START WITH YOUR OWN ONION

GREGORY KELLY

*My dear Michelle
Thank you so much for being part of my life & story
I can't wait to see you
Until then
Love Always
Gregory Kelly May 20*

The events and conversations in this book have been set down to the best of the author's ability.

© Gregory Kelly 2020

All rights reserved. No part of this book may be reproduced or used in any manner without written permission of the copyright owner except for the use of quotations in a book review.

First Edition February 2020

Cover design by Raymond Zada
Back cover portrait "Greg's Eyes" by Grant Burford, 2006

ISBN 978-0-6487821-0-0 (paperback)
ISBN 978-0-6487821-1-7 (ebook)

Published by Gregory Kelly

PREFACE

It was mentioned that I needed to correct all the different measurements into one standard measurement. I say to that: I have had to decipher everything from Nana Young's old world handwriting to modern groovy chefs who believed in a splash of this and a sprinkle of that or the precision chefs who add 3.5 grams of this and 7.2 grams of that, which is a mind-numbingly dull way of cooking for a family!

The thing is, with the recipes mentioned in this collection, some refer to a harvest of things. So fruit from friends' trees for jams, or olives to be cured or even a score at the reduced aisle of the supermarket - these are mainly processes with a bit of calculation. An example being: I love to go to the Adelaide Central Market. Over summer, strawberries get marked down and I can never resist spending a few hours, over two days, making jam. I've been known to have ten kilos of jam cooking away. I know I can't eat that much but family and friends get a bounty as presents. So I am giving you a broad table that will try and accommodate.

When converted, some recipes seem distorted in a way; they sort of lose their authenticity, so I have left them as

PREFACE

they are. Nana Young's Christmas cake, written in her handwriting, is in pounds. It just looks out of place in kilos.

I think one of my dear friends Peter had the right idea when he said: I'm not going to patronise you, you're all intelligent, work it out for yourselves darlings!

* * *

Measurements

1 teaspoon – pretty self-explanatory
1 tablespoon – between 15 to 20mls
1 cup – about 250gms
1 fluid cup – between 200 and 250mls
1 ounce of flour – two level tablespoons – around 30gms
1 ounce of butter – 1 tablespoon
1 pound "lb" – approximately 500gms
"A few" – between 3-5 or 6 dependant on the volume of what you're making

Oven temperatures

Hot means at least 200c to 220c
A moderate oven is anywhere between 165c to 180c
A slow or low oven is 120c to 150c
A cool oven generally under 130c.

The thing with stove tops, ovens and any sort of cooking implement is they are all different! So if you're working on an unfamiliar stove, you need to be aware that some ovens have two temperatures: hot and off. What you know as 180c on yours may not necessarily be the same on another. I know that sounds dumb, but there are a million factors as to why there would be differences; from the oven seal on the door to a faulty temperature gauge. A lovely fan-forced oven

PREFACE

is a great thing to cook with, but they aren't in every house you might find yourself cooking in. The golden rule for every oven is check what you put in it a bit more than usual if you're doing it for the first time.

These are just a guide. In baking I have found you can be a little out; a little here a little there – it's not a devastating problem. Does it really matter that the chocolate chip cookies are a little firm? Firm cookies are great for dunking, crumbly cookies are great for cheesecake crusts. The important thing is they're homemade cookies and they taste great. I try not to admit defeat whatever the outcome!

I remember once making a birthday cake for my brother Paul. One little problem was when I doubled the recipe I forgot to double the flour. It looked great while it was baking, but as I took it out of the oven it collapsed and fell to about 2cms high. When it was cool I put it in the freezer. Then once it became really firm I sliced it through twice getting three layers and with chocolate sauce, strawberries and lots of cream, we had a birthday cake and it was okay, just very fudgy if I remember rightly. So unless its burnt, don't freak out – enjoy the experience! Food is the ultimate seducer xx.

* * *

The Tablespoon

I love and have generally always used an old fashioned tablespoon. I have two with "McQ" engraved on them. These come from the McQuade's; Dad's side of the family who owned or ran several pubs from the 20's to the 60's, including the Esplanade Hotel in St Kilda.

Tot McQuade, Nana Kelly's cousin, had some arrangement with Nana Kelly, where Nana was a servant of Tot's.

PREFACE

Nana spent a lot of Dad's childhood in Dandenong working at the Albion Hotel in the dining room. During this time Dad saw Nana once every two weeks or so and was brought up mainly by his two aunts and his rather austere sounding grandfather. This grandfather was known for sitting a naughty child on the stove for punishment, burning the child's legs. Not the friendliest chap I'm led to believe.

One of the most intriguing things about Dad for me is that he had virtually no strong male role models as a child. His father abandoned Cath Kelly (Dad's mother) when Dad was about 18 months old. Dad remembers seeing him once at about 10 years old. He never saw or wanted to see him. In fact, he was vehement about never wanting to see or find him. In the early years of their marriage, Mum always thought he'd arrive one day at the front door. He never did.

When Tot went to God she had no offspring. By command of her father's will, significant wealth went to the local Catholic church. That particular parish had a significant number of child abuse claims in Victoria with a particular heinous number of crimes committed.

* * *

The Sharpest Knife in the Drawer

As a child, for some reason lost to time, I seemed to have a fascination with electricity. Once whilst on a family holiday in Yarram on a farm my brother Paul said to me "Put your hand on the wire fence and see what happens."

I was a bit gullible and realised I'd been set up when my hand froze for a second or two as I grasped the wire. It was electric of course, and hurt (scared me more, embarrassed me even more), though some of the others thought it was funny. Happy day, that one!

Another time found me in the laundry with a plug that had only about 20cm of cord ending in exposed wires. I thought it might be interesting to plug it in and as the wires touched I flew across the laundry.

The third time was the last. It involved me trying to get the plug of the toaster out of the socket. It seemed to be wedged in there so I thought I'd grab a stainless steel knife and try and pry it out. And again I flew! This time across our kitchen, which was a much bigger room than the laundry, and a much further flight!

The end result of this little experiment was the sharpest knife ever. It used to be a butter knife with a round head on the blade. After that incident, it had what appeared to be two teeth marks cut out of the round edge. The blade itself must have exploded because it went from a blunt edge to almost a serrated or jagged edge. It never needed sharpening and cut through just about anything. The knife lives on to this day but has lost its sharpness over time. This must have happened over 45 years ago when I was about five or six. Gregory's knife, as it was known in the family, was the sharpest knife in the drawer.

INTRODUCTION

If I ruled the world, real estate agents, anybody in the car selling game, and basically all forms of advertisers would be banned from using adjectives. In particular, advertising of pharmaceuticals and real estate, in my observation, have bastardised language to the point of many adjectives becoming meaningless.

"Greatest views", "may have side effects", "super- food", "one in a million", "state of the art", "nutritious" and my biggest gripe is anything to do with the word "perfection", especially around food.

The idea of perfection in life generally is ridiculous and therefore that would apply to cooking. The only person that has the capacity to say it honestly to you is you. It's when you've done something a few times and, of the times you've done it, one in particular stands out for you. By getting a bit adventurous swapping around flavours and tastes in a recipe, each end result will generally have subtle to extreme end results. They're all good, but once in a while when the end result passes the taste, mouth feel, texture and aroma

INTRODUCTION

tests it can be a little thrill; when the cooking gods conspire to create fabulous. Such moments for me are as follows:

- A 40th birthday pressie to me from Shane and Neil. We were in Kakadu National Park. Steaks bought in Humpty Doo, cooked on an open fire with boiled potatoes with a blast of pesto. The setting and company was unforgettable, the menu was relatively simple (meat and spuds), but such beauty was in that meal and surroundings.
- Joanne arriving whilst I was losing weight rapidly during the mid 90's and stocking the cupboards with all sorts of goodies which we feasted upon for a week. My heart and body got some rejuvenation with delicious foods, hugs and laughter.
- Getting taken out for lunch or dinner and just being treated to an abundance. I love every meal ever cooked for me.
- Liza rocking up with amazing champagnes on many occasions and having wonderful afternoons of bubbles and nibbly bits.
- Making fudge and being unsuccessful, getting a crystallised end result the few times I attempted, but on the third try getting a lovely rich creamy texture.
- Cooking the flourless chocolate cake having a few less than fabulous end results and then getting it just right. This means a look and touch of a sponge with the mouth feel and taste of a chocolate mousse. Pretty damn sexy!

INTRODUCTION

- Mum and my seven-layered Pavlova at Dad's 80th. I will say that was a triumph.
- When Emmanuel comes to stay and I can hand over my kitchen and let him cook.
- Belle's toffee crusted, chocolate, fruit damper cooked in the fire pit at Confest.

A hard lesson in my life has been to look myself in the mirror and feel good about myself – let alone perfect. Accepting myself for who I am, what my life is, how I've behaved to myself and others have been huge tasks. Now I try to use this knowledge not to waste a minute of life. I think back on those occasions and I'm humbled for a moment – and honoured to have sat in amongst and receive perfection. They have been somewhat magic moments, each one of them.

What is my self-esteem; my self-image? For me it is what I make it. If I "feed" it crap it will live, to a point. In the same respect, if I "feed" it the best I can, I believe I can live better.

Most of the cooking media I see profess the highest quality and generally that means the most expensive cut of meat, spice, farinaceous oddity or vegetable that is out of season and flown around the world with a huge carbon footprint. This clamouring for an ultimate thrill at an extraordinary expense doesn't deal with many of today's society's eating issues. That is another gripe I have; when it comes to food and cooking, Australia is fast becoming a fat country. The idea of putting people into unfamiliar situations, no apparent skills (according to the advertising) and creating incredibly stressful scenarios with an expectation of success I think is very counter-productive to the viewer (or eater) who

INTRODUCTION

wants to eat well and keep relatively healthy. Televised competitions, I believe, want to show the audience that, for incredible amounts of anguish, you too can serve up a meal that looks and probably tastes restaurant quality. But at what cost in emotion, time, effort and dollars? I believe all this really does is send a message of "eating well is expensive, laborious and far too complicated for anyone to do – especially me!"

Following a labour-intensive recipe requires a few definite skills like time-management and focus skills. But really, does the average person have the time to eat to this standard daily? The real skill I believe is being able to look at a pantry or refrigerator and put something together with what you can see. Always be respectful of the ingredients, try not to burn it, make it because you want to eat something satisfying, hopefully make something that has a certain health focus (relative to the situation of opening someone else's pantry), and to have an enjoyable experience with loved ones or strangers. If there's enough left over, some can be frozen for times when you just want a quick meal.

Starting with an onion is always the first step for me. Any onion will do and by that I'm including spring, white, brown, red, leek, garlic or any powdered garlic or onion you can grab. A general rule is to sweat/sauté your onions when cooking. So find an onion, pot, knife, oil, stove and you are off and running. On a low to moderate heat, chopped onions in a pot with some olive oil slowly cooking without too much colour is sweating or sautéing.

Many times I've had people ask me "How can you walk into an unfamiliar place and just whip up a meal?"

In my life so far, I seem to have been in many situations where cooking a simple meal, for as many as required, has been uplifting and healing. When depression, illness or death cause situations where cooking is too hard, to be able to assist a relative, friend or stranger at these times in life is truly rewarding. It doesn't have to be a three-course meal. Cooking laden with stress is never fun.

The side effects I've experienced with being HIV positive for well over two decades have been mainly centred on food going in and staying in, until it reaches the other destination, in the most beneficial way. Food, family and friends have been integral to why I'm here and healthy, looking at older age.

When the side effects did take hold and keeping food in was almost impossible, even a slice of lemon in warm water was a luxury. To be able to clean my mouth and keep some moisture in my body was an indulgence close to perfection!

To all those who have nourished my body and soul. Mum, Nana Young, Shane, Emmanuel, Joanne, Grant, Uncle Dave, Augustina and Clement, who I know have cooked for me probably hundreds to thousands of times. To everybody that has ever cooked a meal for me, I give thanks to you for preparing and serving it with love xx.

ONE
PRECURSORS TO A METHOD

I have walked and talked with, loved, and am loved by Angels.

That statement might sound like a new-age thing to say. It may sound as if I've discovered some fundamentalist, pseudo-Christian God force who is determined to get retribution and will send me to the pits of hell given half a chance if I don't conform. Let me allay your fears; it has nothing to do with any concept, dogma, or theory. It doesn't involve suspending rationale, scientific research or aligning your chakras with your reiki force field. It certainly won't challenge those of you who are religious. For you, maybe my stories could be confirmation of a god. Or not. I don't know. I do know I have to write this to acknowledge some of the more life-challenging things that have happened to me. In doing this, I gain a sense of amazement at my life and the fact I have a story to tell. I believe in the healing therapy of sharing our stories. Consider this my contribution to sharing, and if my story is worth telling I'm sure you'll let me know. Honesty is paramount in families and cooking.

I'm in extraordinary health, feeling loved, respected, and astounded that I am here!

* * *

My 50th birthday whizzed by in 2015. Saying that I'm 50 years old actually makes me smile. I really hadn't planned for this to happen.

After being HIV positive for well over 20 years, being told at age 27 (in 1993) that I had six months to two years left of my life, having felt I'd lived through a war, losing so many friends, suffering significant mental health issues, a heart attack and all manner of side effects from medication, even car accidents; I'm still here …

* * *

Nana Young's Quince Jam and Paste

- Wipe the quinces well
- Do not peel; cut fruit into pieces
- Put in to a pan with water enough to cover them
- Boil until soft
- Pass through a sieve, discard the leftover peelings
- Then weigh the strained fruit to every pound add 1lb of sugar
- Boil till firm and rich in colour

My method:

When it comes to quinces I believe in squeezing every lovely morsel out of the fruit. Not to contradict Nana, but if you have a lot of quinces I find it easier to peel and core them. By boiling up the scraps you maximise the fruit and capture the pectin that sets the end result.

- Put the scraps, cores and peel into one pot and the fruit into another
- Cover with water and boil till the liquid is a ruby colour and fruit is soft
- Strain the scraps and liquid, discard scraps and set aside liquid
- This liquid can either be used making quince jelly or alternatively adding to the boiled quinces.

Going back to Nana Young's recipe:

- The fruit pulp needs to be weighed, so let it cool if it's hot. Once it's weighed you add the same amount of sugar
- Also it's a good idea to put the cool fruit in a food processor, puree then combine with the sugar in the cooking pot
- Add some lemon juice to taste depending on the tartness of quinces
- Cook the mixture on high for a few minutes stirring with a wooden spoon till the sugar has dissolved, then turn the heat down low and cook till it's thick and ruby in colour – this can take an hour or two dependant on the volume of

fruit you started with. You don't need to stand over it but check it every 5-10 minutes
- For quince jam cook fruit till you get a good colour and set a teaspoon of mixture on a plate that's been in the freezer or at least cold (think Melbourne winter) and if it's cooked enough it will set, which means it won't run over the plate. It is a visual thing (or spend a few dollars buy a jam and candy thermometer)
- For quince paste, which I prefer, you need to cook it down further – it will appear to come away from the sides of the pot when it's ready
- With the liquids the fruit and scraps were boiled in, for every 4 cups of liquid add 3 cups of sugar and some lemon juice and reduce till candy thermometer says 'jelly stage'. This makes quince jelly and is fabulous on scones or anything where jam is used.

* * *

My Nana (Mum's mum), Annie Young, was born in 1900. She was a granddaughter of Albert Millman, reported through family history to be the oldest surviving member of the Eureka Stockade. A photograph hangs in the Ararat Historical Society taken in 1918 for the town's Diamond Jubilee. Albert was part of a group of people collectively called the "Pioneers of Ararat". Apparently he spoke several languages, including French, and was often called upon to translate letters for various dignitaries in his community. He went on to have 11 children and is buried in Ararat Cemetery. Mum, Dad and I met up in Ballarat for the weekend in November 2018. My dear friend Letho Kostoglou, who was the first Australian to complete the Requiem in Mozart's traditional style (as Mozart died before he completed it), had invited us to be guests of honour at its premiere at St Paul's Cathedral. I'd come from Adelaide and Mum and dad had taken the train from Melbourne. Before driving them home on the Sunday I took them to Ararat Cemetery where we found Albert's grave (we think) – a solid slab and name plate which just says "Millman" with no other identification on it.

Annie's husband, Donald (Don) Patrick Campbell Young, was too young to fight in WWI and worked on the railways, which were called "essential services", during the Second War. He had a brother who fought and died on the Western Front in 1916 in France during the First World War. His body was never found. Don passed away on Boxing Day 1975. Mum and Dad and all six kids were visiting to help eat the leftovers from Christmas Day. He had mowed the lawn and weeded the vegetable garden. He went into his bedroom and had a massive heart attack. I'll never forget Annie screaming *'Don, don't leave me Don! Don't leave me!'*

Annie and Don had five children. The eldest son, Allan, went to the Second World War. He met his future wife Pam when they were both assigned to the *Special Wireless Group* where they helped intercept Japanese Army and Navy radio messages this included a stint in New Guinea. Both Allan and Pam took down the Japanese Kana in Morse code, then passed that information through the chain of command. They both received the Bletchley Park Medal after 50 years of sworn secrecy, which included getting a citation from UK Prime Minister Gordon Brown. When they returned from war, Allan continued his career as a school teacher and they had four children. Pam was an avid dog lover and later in life set up a boarding kennel in Benalla.

Nancy, Annie and Don's second child, was a complex woman. She was deserted by her husband with two small children in the early 1950's. I remember visiting her in 1992 in Maroubra, Sydney, where she had lived for many years. The day before I had visited Allan and Pam who gave me some tomatoes to give to Nancy. She was really delighted that these were tomatoes from her brother's garden. On a visit several years later she proudly showed me the plants she had grown from the seeds from her brother's tomatoes. Benalla is a 700km drive from him to her.

Shelia was the third child, another complex woman who married Alan Morrison. For Mum's early life Shelia was one of Mum's closest friends. I never really knew Shelia all that well. She was a bit outrageous (as an adult I realise she had mental health issues that were never really talked about). Shelia and Alan had three children.

Next there was Mum, followed seven years later by the fifth child: Michael, who Annie had at the age of 49. Michael married Norma, my favourite aunt (I think this could possibly be due to the fact that she was the most contemporary in age to my siblings and I). They had three children, who were our closest relations growing up.

Collectively, at the time of her death, Annie and Donald had 18 grandchildren. Today they would have great, great grandchildren. Annie loved cooking and eating, loved being the hostess, and loved feeding people. There was always food in the cupboard in case visitors dropped by. A meal could be served in no time, according to Mum. I remember jars of boiled lollies in the cupboard and home-made biscuits, huge Christmas lunches or dinners for what felt like hundreds of people.

A sort of tradition or cultural ritual between Annie and her elder sister Jo during big family gatherings was: *As long as the men are fed!* Mum remembers this with a touch of animosity because as a child she had to wait till all the men were served, who were in the lounge room with racing forms not doing anything. They missed out on the beautiful smells from all the smoking they were doing.

I remember sitting with Annie in the hospital in 1982, when I was 15 years old. I was holding her hand. Annie loved clothes, makeup and relished entertaining. She was always so exuberant, but in that moment, in hospital, she was virtually lifeless, the machines attached to her beeping away. She had been in hospital for some 18 hours. Our younger brother Matthew found her on the floor in her home. He and Mum had gone to check on her when Nana couldn't be contacted. They ended up breaking a window to get into the house and Matthew, a small boy, crawled through. He discovered her and opened the front door to let Mum in. She'd had a massive stroke.

Mum and the rest of the family spent almost all the time she had left by her side. I recall going home for about an hour during that period. I knew Nana was dying. I loved her so much and I just wanted to be with her. Her breathing was incredibly laboured. If you've ever heard that type of breathing before you'll know what I am talking about; long drawn out rattle sounds emanated from this once vibrant, loving and now unconscious woman. I had been holding and gently stroking her hand for a long time and we had fallen into the rhythm of her breathing. Then, with a bit of a splutter, she slightly opened her left eye which appeared to give a wink. Her mouth on her left side moved slightly into a smile. She gave my hand the tiniest squeeze, and then she was gone.

This experience has never left me. Being such a gracious exit, I have no particular fear about dying. The process ... I am not too keen on.

* * *

I came out to my parents individually, about eight months apart. I expected the fury of religious dogma to turn me out of the house of my childhood. I was fully prepared to be evicted.

At first, Mum was concerned about how the rest of the family would take it, but they already knew. Her fears of rejection by them were unfounded. I do remember her saying, surprised: *'Even the priest knows!'*

I explained that I had gone to confession and was advised by the priest that it wouldn't be a good thing if I told them. Mum found a letter in the cupboard of the bedroom that the four of us boys had shared. It was a letter I wrote to myself when I was about 14 and forgotten about. I was working at Queenscliff Hotel and was home for my days off when she confronted me about this letter.

'Are you a homosexual?'

'Yes,' was my reply. We spoke for a long time. Mum advised me to not to tell Dad for a while, as his mother was dying at the time. She had been in hospital having had her legs removed from diabetes related issues (which I thought was obscene at 90 years old).

So I waited for a few months after Nana Kelly had died and prepared the family; I was going to tell Dad. We arranged a time (for the only time in our lives, everyone arrived on time) and the family gathered to help Dad with the news. I will always be very proud of them. Dad cried,

START WITH YOUR OWN ONION

hugged me and said: '*I don't care who you sleep with. You are still my son and I love you.*'

This reaction (even today, some 30 years later) is not a common reaction. It's more likely that the prejudices and intolerance will come marching out. I choose to believe that Nana Young was helping Mum and Dad during this time.

It was not long after this I recall reading a headline in the newspaper: *Gay Plague Hits Australia*. I had been going out to gay pubs and nightclubs when I noticed the first signs of men who had "IT". "IT" being a look. The look physically said "I have IT"; sunken faces, thinning bodies, dark red stains on the skin (Kaposi's sarcoma) and downcast eyes. No one knew what "IT" was but soon enough we were to see its onslaught.

At about 24, when some of my closer friends began to suffer and die, Mum, Dad and I started to volunteer at a place called *St Francis House*; a halfway house for people living with HIV who also had drug and alcohol issues. It was actually one of the first of its kind in the world.

The first friend I knew to die was more a close friend of Mum and Dad's, John, who started the house with his partner Steve, and a group of nuns from the Daughters of Charity order.

These were the days when there was little to no information surrounding HIV; no drugs, no knowledge on prevention, nothing to stop it. I call this time *"The War Years"*. We were all soldiers trying to alleviate the pain and shame, and buffer some of the intolerance of the rest of society.

My very brave and extraordinary parents worked with men who were gay, dying, who had been sex workers, or just had had lots of sex, or just sex once, intravenous drug users, men who had been in jail, trans persons. Some were very effeminate, some not. There was a ballet dancer from a major Australian ballet company, men who basically had no one or nowhere to go – other than St Francis House. My parents, Margaret and Vincent, were surrogate parents for many amazingly diverse men around the time of their deaths.

Around my 27th birthday I only had one or two gay long-term friends left in Melbourne. I had buried approximately 50 of them including several lovers, many friends, and well-respected people. The pain was intolerable. There were times when I was invited to weddings and christenings and if a funeral wasn't on the same day, it was the next.

I had to leave Melbourne and start afresh. I travelled to Byron Bay and started my own business. Just under a year later I was given the diagnosis of being HIV positive. I asked the doctor what he believed my outlook was. His response was that if I didn't go onto AZT (one of the first antiretrovirals) immediately I would have six months to two years to live. I laughed at such a suggestion. It was possibly more out of fright than humour, but I said: 'So you are telling me that I won't get hit by a bus in the next six months?'

To me, AZT had been associated with more deaths than people it had helped. I refused to take it. We know now it was overprescribed. In defence of these actions, it seemed no one really had any idea what they were treating. I consider all my friends who took it to be guinea pigs. Much more than that, they were martyrs. Without their sacrifice I would not be here today – nor would HIV/AIDS be considered a chronic, manageable illness, which it is today.

Death and grief continued to ride the wave of sick men in Byron Bay and the Northern Rivers. I had become close friends with a man called Max (he was close with everyone he met, including Mum and Dad). He'd been diagnosed in

START WITH YOUR OWN ONION

the late stages of the viral attack. I chose to become one of his carers. I knew him alive for 18 months. Max had major body breakdown and it was only a short time before he left us; his immunity to any disease was virtually gone.

One particular day I had been given the day off in caring for him. Martin, another close friend of Max, was a strong man and offered to care for him. He met me at the door and said: 'Good morning! You're having a day off. Go to the beach and chill.' I followed his advice.

Before the beach, I went in and said my hellos to Max. 'That'll be right! Leave me by myself!' He said in a soft but very camp, theatrical, mocking way. I left laughing.

Brays Beach, surrounded by the beautiful Broken Head National Park, was a short bike ride away from Max's. It was here on this day that something happened. In trying to describe what happened, words don't fit. I was the only person on the beach. I sat in a yoga posture, legs crossed, and closed my eyes. On my own at the beach, I just sat there and felt the sea breeze on my face. I remember "seeing", with eyes closed, the beautiful horizon of blues, the waves rolling in, the foam, birds flying ... then, Nana Young stepped out as clear as day and said: 'Hello dear. Are you looking after yourself?'

She was followed by my grandfather (Don) who asked the same question. Six other dead friends appeared along with Nana Kelly, all questioning me, wanting to know if I was looking after myself. They all seemed to sit around me and I'm not sure entirely of the conversation other than being asked the question: *Are you looking after yourself?*

I remember turning my head and seeing a light camel colour, the same colour of Max's couch where he spent most of his time. In this colour was a pencil cartoon of Max moving as if he was caught in a web or some sort of glue. His long, thin arms and legs appeared weighed down by the force of whatever he was caught in. 'Max!' I remember saying, shocked at what I was seeing.

Nana Young was in front of me saying: 'Don't worry about Max, darling. We are all looking after him. He is fine. It is you that has to look after yourself.'

There were more things that happened. For lack of a better description, it was a dream-state, but incredibly powerful for me.

It was late afternoon by the time I had the energy to move. I wasn't sure of what had happened, but the knowledge that so many people were looking after my dear friend was so overwhelmingly beautiful. It was such a comfort. Dead people had always been separate from the living in my head (bizarre as that sounds). This was the first moment in my life when both the living and dead had been in the same conversation. Whatever happened, I felt an incredible peace start to fill the space in me that had been hollowed out with dread of his dying, and all of my friends dying in such pain.

I went home to find two friends, Shane and Robert, who had not liked each other for as long as I had known them. They were deep in conversation and looked at me, amazed at the fact they did like each other. I thought this symbolic in a way, then I said: 'Well you are not going to believe what's just happened to me.'

I relayed what had happened and when I finished the beach story I added: '... and to come in here, and see you two getting along has blown me away!'

I rang Mum to tell her what had happened. 'I do not know whether it was a dream, a hallucination, or a message from God but Mum ... it has made the fact that Max, who we all know is not long with us, is going to be looked after! It makes it a lot easier.'

It was about a week later when I got the courage to tell Max of what happened. He said: 'You silly poof, you have already told me this.'

'No, this is the first time.'

'Well that must be who they are!' he said

'Who are they, Max?'

'I've had all these people around me for a couple of weeks ... and I didn't know who they were ... A few old folks, bald man, big woman, couple of girls from the 50's, a few queens.'

'Are they ok to you Max?' I asked.

'Oh yeah they're just fine. I just didn't know who they were.'

From that day till he died, as by then the cancers, infections and morphine had taken control, he would say to me: 'I'm so glad you told me who they were.'

There were other things that were said on that day, and they have remained with me. However I try to describe what I saw and heard that day – whether it be hallucination, meditation, visitation or a mini breakdown – it enabled me to share the pain of watching a dear friend's death, and the absolute knowledge that I was powerless over this process.

I choose to believe that I have a posse of relations and friends in another place looking after Max, me, and all of us.

At this stage of his life his mind wandered, but he always knew who I was, and he always knew who they were. He was safe and protected. I can only call this walking with Angels.

* * *

GREGORY KELLY

Shane's Hainan Chicken

- Cover chicken with lightly salted water adding carrot, celery, leek, ginger, garlic, bay leaf
- Bring to boil then gentle poach for 1 hour
- Cook rice in stock and steam some bok choy
- Serve chicken with a bowl of clear chicken stock with finely grated ginger mixed with a little rice vinegar.

* * *

February 2001

I was supposed to be looking after Mum following a hysterectomy. I was supposed to be cooking for Dad. I was supposed to be helping out.

Driving home from the hospital after leaving Mum, I felt major discomfort in my side. It intensified to the point where it felt like I'd had a golf ball inserted in me. Emanating from my right side above my hip, the pain got so bad over the next couple of hours that Dad took me to the local hospital. I was admitted and it began ...

Nothing will fill me with more horror; send me straight to a denial tantrum than the words "clear fluid diet." When I was told this is what I would be living on, I was in agony; really out of it on doctors' administered pain relief, but I was still in pain, incredibly frightened, depressed, and extremely emotional. Add to this state of mind: guilt about how I had spoken to the young woman who had the unfortunate task of telling me '*I'm sorry Mr. Kelly but the doctor has put you on a Clear Fluid Diet.*' My heart goes out to her now but I have to say: due to the emotional state I was in, she did receive hell-fire from a very upset man.

START WITH YOUR OWN ONION

This was one of those life challenges, one on a list titled *"The Worst, Most Unpleasant Things."* It was the first time I had been aware of having morphine. The nurse came in every once in a while to ask: 'Are you in pain, love?'

I can remember responding 'Oh, sort of,' or something like that, and the response was always: 'OK, we'll just top you up then.'

For three and a half days I knew that I was really not with the *"Conscious Ones."* They're the people that all buzz around you when you're in hospital and you're on the bed; dazed, clinging as if you may fall off. I was under the impression when we arrived at the hospital that the doctors would fix me up and my stay would be an overnight thing. I was secure. I didn't need to eat. I was really out of it.

Mum and Dad came to visit and I recall thinking *I'm whacked off my face in front of my parents* and, in a way, it was sort of cool. Well, as cool as a stay in hospital can get doing heavy duty drugs. No safer place than to have the experts administering them. Not that I think being that out of it is in any way cool. Dribbling mouth and scattered brains – definitely not cool.

I have certainly known many people from all walks of life that have thought of heroin as their heroine, but I have never had the desire. Give me a cold glass of bubbly, Guinness, scotch, beer, vodka or a big fat joint. With alcohol or pot you can see, feel, smell the quality, and you can control the intake. With the magic white powders and pills there ain't no turning back.

I have never had this rather naive trust that some of the party circuit seems to have when it comes to pills and powders. Let's face it: speed kitchens wouldn't have the government health regulations that a brewery has ... and as for home grown marijuana: I do believe God gave it to us for a reason.

The eyes always get to me. Those pinned pupils – or with some other drugs, the fat pupils. The glowing irises are worse than any horror movie because this is reality. I find it challenging sometimes to look into eyes on opioids. In many people all I can see is pain.

The appetite stimulation and anti-nausea effect of my drug of choice, marijuana, are two powerful reasons why it's been important in my life. I realise this was the first use of heavy pain killer medication. I often thought about what my eyes looked like but I wouldn't really have been able to focus in a mirror to see.

If there is one solid comfort in life that I can always rely on it is food. Starting with the Sunday fry-up, Nana's scones with homemade jam and cream, chocolate, roast lamb dinners, the taste and aromas of vegetables or herbs straight from the garden are all things that make me feel good. Whatever it is, solid comfort food is very reliable. I love foods that are nostalgic; connected with some emotion. I believe there are foods that can substitute sex. I've had quite a few mouth orgasms! And the pleasure of being able to play with some really beautiful ingredients. When this basic luxury was taken away from me it felt like the end of the world.

By the second day in hospital I was starting to feel as if someone had stuck me on hold and for some reason I just kept hanging on the telephone. Doctors were undecided as to how or why I was in so much pain and gave me four possibilities, each requiring the removal of organs. It could have been appendix bursting, gall bladder erupting, kidneys failing, or pancreas collapse. Totally bummer news when you are really out of it and hanging out for Nanna to walk around the corner next to your bed with a bowl of chicken soup or fresh scones and jam *'Cos you'll feel better, luv.'* And who wouldn't?

Although I was desperately craving some decent food, in reality one of the symptoms I came to hospital with was vomiting, so I thought: *Whatever the reason I'm here in hospital, I think it's better Nanna stays home, I suppose.* In fact, at that time, Nanna had been buried over 20 years.

I was craving chocolate and I couldn't have it because of a small, magnetic sticker they had put over my bed. The repugnant sticker read *"NIL ORALLY."* I remember thinking: *I'm sure that wasn't there yesterday and does that mean ... what, exactly?* I pushed the call button for the nurse. I was muttering under my breath all sorts of insults about her. I thought I may have waited for a while so whilst I was waiting I started thinking about chocolate. *I need chocolate now. I've got to get up. I'm getting up. I'm going to the kiosk. I'm gonna have chocolate. I have to have chocolate now. Get up. Come on. Oh fuck the tube thing in my arm ... Oh it's on a stand trolley thing. That's gotta come too. Push body, heading toward the door, oh come on, you are on a roll here. Something's not right, something can't figure, what is it? Something ... oh dickhead!* I really thought I was in motion but in fact I hadn't left the bed. I started again. *Get up Gregory. Whoa.* Movement, real movement comes all so slow. *Grab that pole grab, the tube thing. Don't bang your – FUCK!!*

I don't know if I was speaking to myself; whether my mouth was moving or I was just thinking these thoughts. I'm pretty sure I swore loudly when I banged my hand and pulled the tube at the same time. It was more just the visual than the actual pain in a weird, delayed sort of way. It reminded me of giving blood for the three-monthly blood tests. I find it easier not to look. I have to turn away. Never let doctors take blood from you, it will hurt. I always feel safer if a nurse is doing it.

Anyway, one foot on the ground yeah here we go ... next foot yeah it's gonna happen just think chocolate. Two legs poised over the bed, head seems to be at a further distance than normal from my feet. Don't worry, that's just the shit doing funny things to you. Now off the bed, get that forward motion happening! Stand. Shit – I pulled the tube! I got out the wrong side, have to walk around the bed to get the stand. One foot forward. Here we go, come on. It's happening, I'm on a roll here! Closer, closer, getting to the door. I can taste it; that delicious milky taste melting all of this madness away. Slow, tentative steps, holding on to tubes and trolley, out the door. Fuck all these people. Don't look at them, they'll know I'm out of it. Hey this seems a bit six million-dollar man all that slow motion stuff. Don't think anything – just chocolate! It's only two flights down to the kiosk! You're gonna make it! A clear loud voice over my shoulder brings me into the "Conscious Ones" realm.

'Excuse me Mr. Kelly, Greg?'
Oh shit, sprung! 'Who, me?'
'Where are you off to, love?'
'I want chocolate'
'Sorry dear, you can't have that'
'I'm going to cry.'
'And then you'll vomit, love, and I'll have to clean it up.'

I could see the sense in her argument, and boy, did I feel like an argument ... so I muttered 'bitch' under my breath.

'Pardon?'
'I've got an itch.'
'I understand. Come on let's get back to bed. You might have to be operated on today. Are you in pain?'

'Sort of ...'
'On a scale of one to ten, if ten is the worst?'
'Seven.'
'Oh. I'll get the doctor.'
More fucking morphine! Not sure I like this shit.

Sometime later – it could have been five minutes, it could have been several hours – a short, Asian man, maybe in his late forties, with a thick accent starts looking at me.

His mouth is moving. I wonder if he is talking to me. He is looking at me. I suppose he is. What's he saying, I wonder? I'd better listen.

'Sorry, I wasn't paying attention. Can you repeat what you've just said?' I asked.

'I am your doctor. Do you want to know what's wrong with you?'

'Of course I do, it's just the morphine makes my mind wander.'

'I'll start again.' He then proceeded to waffle on about my kidney; telling me I must have had a bad diet and drank a lot and that I may need it removed.

I responded to him with all the energy that I could muster: 'You think it's the kidney? The other guy said he was definite it was my pancreas.' *Or did he? Maybe he said appendix. But this is new: two doctors, different scare-tactics.*

'I'm the specialist here, I make the decisions. Do you want my opinion or not? As I said at the start – but you weren't listening – we are still unsure what is wrong. I do believe this, so we may operate today.'

'Does that mean I still can't eat?'

'No eating.'

With that, he disappeared through the doorway, amongst all the Conscious Ones. *I really want chocolate now. Did he have attitude or what? Are they going to take out my kidneys and pancreas? I want Mum and Dad and chocolate!*

'Has the doctor seen you, love?'

'Who?' I asked.

'The doctor'

'I dunno.'

'Well sweetheart, we have to give you a clean out – an enema. Just lie on your side. That's right, knees up. A little higher. That's it.'

Into me she squirts. *The irony,* I think to myself

'Now hold on as long as you can and when you go to the loo you have to call the nurse and show her what you've done.'

'I beg your pardon?' *I mean, how much reality do you need?*

Time slipped by as the fluid did what it was supposed to do. I waited for as long as possible. I suppose it was the thought of losing all this fluid; that – as confused as I was – I still didn't need to embarrass myself. I hurled my body through the mental haze. This time on the right side of the bed, stabled myself on the pole, and headed across the hallway to the toilet. There I sat to let gravity take its course.

I startled myself a little while later when a pool of dribble started to run onto my thigh. I wiped my mouth and pushed the call button. I was building up to another life challenge, in other words: one of the more humiliating moments of my life. A very unfriendly face opened the door and demanded to know what I wanted in a loud, assertive way.

'I've been told that I have to show you this,' I replied.

This woman didn't win any brownie points when she threw open the door, so I lost my embarrassment quite instantly and lifted myself up. I knew from her face that she wasn't relishing this either.

'Yeah, okay. I'll mark it down.'

Needless to say, I didn't share any more of these moments with the nurses. I just took my own mental notes when these overwhelming urges took hold.

In the morning, when the ward started pumping back to life, a nurse entered the room and said: 'Mr. Kelly?' The specialist will see you in about half an hour. Are you in pain?'

'Sort of.'

I lifted myself up to tell her I didn't like what the morphine was doing to me and uttered: 'Please don't give me–' as my mouth was moving she was putting the drug into my drip. 'I don't like this shit!' I snarled, but faded into la-la land.

She looked at me with shock, then responded: 'Mr. Kelly, the specialist will see you in half an hour. No need to worry.'

It was a little while after the rush, mellow feeling you get from the morphine, and into the semi-hallucinating stage when a tall, pompous, dark-suited man stood at the foot of my bed. I can't remember his name, but he was an arrogant arse that really didn't pay attention to all the facts – actually, none of the five doctors did.

'Now, I've just seen your x-rays, but I just can't see what the problem is. You see, in all my working years I've never seen a bowel so full before, and because your full bowel blocks our view we will have to try and empty you and then go for more tests.'

This was so unexpected and confusing so I asked: 'The HIV medication I'm on has given me phenomenal diarrhoea for years. How could I possibly be constipated?'

'You can have constipation and diarrhoea at the same time.'

'Well, I suppose that doesn't make too much sense, but you're the expert – and you think it's my gall bladder?'

'Yes. But when we clean you out we'll see.'

Many times in my life I have been told - that I am full of shit. But this was the first time someone had the proof to back up that statement.

'So I'll be having more tests and enemas?'

'Yes. I'll see you tomorrow.'

'Can I eat something if I'm not going to be operated on?'

'Just clear fluids, Mr. Kelly.' With that he was gone, off to torture more out-of-it souls.

The last bits of reality came and went as the drug took over. It didn't seem to ever take the pain away, but it came on like a new, rather less interesting dimension. It was a bit like unreality becoming reality. Aretha Franklin and Ray Charles with the Southern Baptist Choir and I were singing rousing gospel tunes with lots of alleluias and Amen's – with the occasional *'Praise the Lord!'* thrown in for good measure. I had a slight feeling this wasn't happening, but I'd never been in such company. Real or unreal, it couldn't be bad. I felt they were with me and I was preparing to go on to glory.

* * *

Another of the Conscious Ones in a white coat came into the room, but not to see me. He sat on the bed of a man named George, who was next to me. George was an old man and was further up the glory ladder than me. He was deaf as a post and tired. Really tired. The doctor proceeded

START WITH YOUR OWN ONION

to loudly ask: 'Are you still depressed? Do you still want to commit suicide? Why did you want to kill yourself?'

Ray, Aretha and the gospel singers all hit the road. I was thrown onto the footpath of Reality Central. I remember my eyes opening, knowing I was hearing the innermost thoughts of an unhappy old man. I was mad; mad at that doctor – no class. Nurses came and spoke to George without having to bellow and got their message across. I couldn't see why this doctor was so arrogant to a clearly broken man. Anyway, I wasn't going to listen. No way. *I have to move tube and trolley, let's get out of here.*

I slowly shuffled to the corridor with the doctor's words still ringing in my ears. At the entrance to the hallway I could see the nurse's station across from me – and the long corridor. *I can't go to the nurses. They'll just put me back into bed.*

Framed prints of different scenes covered the walls of the corridor. One of a young lad in a field of flowers flying a kite, his dog at his side and mountains in the background. It caught my eye. I thought to myself: *That there is where I want to be.* I proceeded to drift into that land of coloured kites and flowers. I faced the print and began to nod off. Sometime later I felt something touch my shoulder.

'What are you doing out of bed?'

'I refuse to listen to the private suicidal thoughts of an old man. It's so undignified and really uncool.'

She knew what I was talking about, as you could still hear the doctor shouting his stupid questions to George. Maybe it was the drugs that magnified the effect, but I hated that doctor intensely.

'Quick, get him a chair,' I heard. My legs felt a bit wobbly. Truth be told, I was probably swaying all over the place. Someone helped me into a chair, still in front of the boy with the kite, and placed a blanket over my lap.

'Do not move from here, just wait till the doctor goes and then it's back to bed.'

Actually, I had no intention of moving from there, as the field of beautiful flowers beckoned me to just go for a walk through it all.

'Come on, back to bed. The silly bugger has gone now there is no more screaming. You won't be forced to hear anything.' So back to bed I went to receive dinner; a bitter-tasting drink that was part of another enema. *After this, I just might get some real dinner – clear fluid, of course.*

Mum and Dad came in to visit to find me neurotic and working myself up into hysterics.

'I think I'm going to die,' I told them.

'Don't talk like that darling, we're here. You'll be all right; they will get to it.

Everyone sends their love. We've had so many phone calls from people asking about you.' Mum proceeded to roll off a list of names, which was really touching and comforting. 'Now, Rosie and Jenny both asked when is a good time to come and visit.'

'No visitors. I don't think I could cope.' I'm not into visitors when I'm in pain. I feel I don't behave well; I'm rude, nasty and usually feel like I'm going to rip someone's arm off. 'I'll see them when I get out. You do think I'm getting out, don't you? Please tell me I'm getting out.' I began to plead with Mum as if she knew something I didn't.

'Of course you are, darling. As soon as you are fixed up. You'll be fine.'

* * *

I know one thing about this life that I have led: I am one of the lucky ones. I may never have had a real partner in life, but I do have what so many gay men don't have and that is loving parents.

During so many funerals between 1989 and 1996 (I did lose count after 80), I saw mothers and fathers standing over their sons' graves full of hate. Hating what their son was, hating what their son had died of, and hating those who had come to mourn. Most of the parents and families didn't know these weird strangers; these friends of the deceased. You could see on their faces: *Which one of these freaks gave this to my son?*

I never understood them at all; these families that had disowned their children because of gayness. I certainly will never understand the notion that you can have a child and only love them if they adhere to some unwritten standards. I remember my dear friend Max. His parents showed up a week before he died. Only once before had his mother visited whilst Max was ill. When he did pass away, his father walked out of Max's room (his body not even cold), into the lounge room and said: 'What the fucking hell are we going to do with all this shit?'

Max's father went on a mental list of people I hate. The "shit" he was referring to was Max's baby grand piano, leather couches, antique furniture and many other fabulous pieces of art. Blinded by the hate and disappointment of who and what his son was, he couldn't even focus on the fact that his own flesh and blood had just died. Maybe now, 20 years later (if he is still alive), he may realise just what he missed out on: being part of his son's life.

That's why I'm so fortunate; I have the acceptance and love of my parents and family. From being a cocky teenager to being in hospital, my parents never despised me. They were there, holding my hand, comforting me, with a probable AIDS-related condition. They have been unbreakable walls of strength and love.

Family secrets are on Mum's side of the family, with dates being changed on wedding certificates. On Dad's side, all documentation relating to Dad's father disappears after 1936. The only photo of Dad's parents' wedding shows the groom and a heavily pregnant bride. Why she would keep that photo in particular seems unusual to me, as she destroyed everything else. Not a trace of Claude Leslie Kelly (or Leslie Claude Kelly, it's unclear what his real name was) could been found. He disappeared after 1936. Lots of issues were buried in the past and never spoken about.

Mum and Dad defied any prejudice and blind Catholic faith was pretty much shattered with two incidents; two events insignificant on a world scale, but major on a family scale. Margaret and Vincent went from Perry Como to Grace Jones with the arrival of grandchild number one and, in the same year, an out homosexual son.

Their reactions showed to me that love can conquer ignorance. I suppose Mum and Dad were so safe with their religion that they didn't need to question any of the doctrines until those doctrines challenged their own children. They are proud people, but not too proud to question their own values and not so proud they would abandon any of their children. I do love them.

To have them at my side through the dark hours of so many ordeals – so many deaths – is, I believe, why I'm alive. One doesn't need a lover (certainly they help!), but we are born into this world through the actions of our parents. Those actions can help us as functional people, or they can induce us to become closeted or dysfunctional and insecure individuals.

* * *

Back at the hospital, dinner arrived as Mum and Dad said their farewells. Three plastic bowls, each with plastic lids. I was scared to open them but temptation got the better of me and through the morphine haze in my head I lifted the lid on the first bowl to see a clear-ish fluid. My nostrils told me that it was what's affectionately called in the hospitality circles *"Rooster Booster."* It comes in a large tin, is a garish yellow colour and, in my bowl, was not dissolved sufficiently. There were a few lumps floating on top of the water, but most of it sat on the bottom of the bowl. If the chemicals didn't upset my stomach, I was sure the horrible colour would. Hunger pains or not, this stuff wasn't going near my mouth. I'd rather lick a live chicken. The green flaky dried bits caught my imagination and I wondered what they could be. Certainly nothing of an organic nature! I mean, the yellow stuff couldn't be, so why would the green bits have any primary connection to a living thing?

If temptation got me to open the first bowl, I think maybe morbid curiosity is why I opened the others. Bowl number two had another sealed bowl inside it. The label read: *Reconstituted fruit juice from local and imported ingredients.* I felt a sensation that I was quite used to by this point: the old magic dry retch.

I buzzed the nurse. A minute or two later she walked in smiling and I asked her for a cup of tea. I let the black tea settle my stomach before reaching over to lift the lid on the third bowl. Underneath sat a solid square of bright red jelly. Tears started falling from my eyes. I felt betrayed. I was going to die and these arseholes were hastening the process. I visualized myself in the kitchen and sent major voodoo magic to the head chef. These guys weren't chefs, they were economic wankers.

I know that it isn't costly or difficult to make stock, especially considering the life-giving energy that a fresh bowl of stock can provide. The simple, clear, clean flavours of chicken broth compared to the nasty chemical assault on the taste buds that "Rooster Booster" can be is incomparable. One will help your body recover from "dis-ease" (Louise Hay), the other will keep you unwell.

As for the reconstituted juice and jelly; these bastards didn't even know what was wrong with me. I had cravings for chocolate but I didn't get any. I knew if I had the acid from the juice and sugar from the jelly, my stomach would have gone into overdrive. The more I started throwing magic at the chef, the more upset I became. For the first time in a long time I settled on a prayer: *God, you never gave me a boyfriend in this life (so I suppose I had a really good time in my past lives) and it does appear you are taking me to your bosom. If I am going to die, Lord, can't I have at least some tiny morsel of something, please?*

When the nurse came in, I was sobbing uncontrollably. I was going to die and I was not even going to get my last supper. She asked me how my dinner was going then looked into my face. 'What's wrong love? Do you need a hug?'

In amongst sobs I spluttered: 'Have you seen what they call a clear fluid diet?'

'Oh poor love- err- yes, I have.'

'The Rooster Booster hasn't even dissolved.'

She looked at me and with a tissue started to wipe my tears said: 'When did you last eat?'

'Over three days ago.' With that she left saying she'd be

back in a moment. When she returned she told me she'd spoken to the doctor and, because it was eight o'clock, I wasn't going to be operated on tonight, so I could have something light.

'What will it be? We have cheese and tomato on white, or egg and lettuce on white.'

'I think it'll be the cheese and tomato, thanks.'

I've had the extreme pleasure of eating some fabulous pastries and breads in my time. It's even more pleasurable to be there when such things are cooking. The aromas given off during preparation and when they are pulled out of the oven, then left to rest or cool add to the delight of eating. These aromas and tastes can be great foreplay to a romantic interlude! One of the best chefs I've ever worked with created a beautiful crayfish mousseline. It was wrapped in brioche, which was superb. I've eaten brioches, unleavened breads, sweetened, fruited, sourdough, croissant and Danish pastries, homemade pasta, gnocchi, spaztle – and with every combination of meats, be they seared, grilled, fried, baked, roasted or served as terrines and charcuterie; cured meats and fishes, antipasto vegetables of every shape and size, but when Nurse Betty brought in two packaged tomato and cheese sandwiches, I felt as though I had been given a reprieve from death's highway.

Very slowly, I chewed with small tentative mouthfuls. Betty told me she had explained to the doctor I was in a little state, and he let me have them. Seeing as it had been three and a half days of not eating I relished the whole eating experience. It certainly was one of those times that make one appreciate not the so-called "finer things" in life, but the simple things. Normally white, soggy sponge bread isn't my bag – especially with tomato, as it tends to go a lot soggier. It didn't matter that it was hermetically sealed, or that it was margarine, plastic cheese and a hard, nearly green tomato – THIS WAS FOOD!

My stomach made noises for ages; loud, rumbling noises that tended to create pain – but it felt good at the same time. I didn't want any morphine, feeling that the sandwiches were going to do a lot more for me health-wise than any painkiller could. Mum had lent me her headphones which I put over my head. I turned on Aretha and the Southern Californian Baptist Choir, pretending that I had just had a bowl of chicken soup with greens and steamed rice. It was one of my favourite meals; a simple broth which is elegant as well as soothing "for all that ails you" and probably one of the most bastardized meals on the planet (other than hamburgers). Such an easy, cheap thing to make and yet the rush to package and condense food into its smallest possible form over the last few decades has, I believe, taken a lot of the life force out of food. It's ironic that this push to condense food was created with the two World Wars. Quoting Spike Milligan: *'Not only are you taken from your homeland, tortured, shot or imprisoned – you are also fed shit. And that was our side.'* How can anyone compare the aroma of a whole chicken or (pieces of chicken: wings, bones, necks) cooking in water, turning the water into life-giving broth, against a tin of bright yellow-coloured salt?

Janis, a co-worker at a hotel I worked at some years ago, had previously worked with a chef who ultimately gave up his restaurants for a television show. I worked in the pastry and dessert section. An extra job that was thrown my way was to make sure all the stocks were made. Although stocks and desserts don't have much in common, I enjoyed making them. It was in Janis's hot entrée section where I had to prepare beef, game, vegetable, fish and chicken stocks. Huge 20 and 30 litre stockpots had to go on as soon as I started work. If I was really organised I would have chopped and prepared the six or seven kilos of onions, carrots and celery the night before. This combined mixture of chopped veggies is called a "mirepoix". Half of the mirepoix had to be roasted off to add to the game and beef stocks. This vegetable mixture was divided up into five pots. Every chef has their own eccentricities about how stocks are to be made. I have had to suffer some fools and their peculiar habits regarding the making of stocks (I believe the only golden rule is: don't boil the fuck out of it).

Janis and I were having a laugh at some of the stories we recalled when she said: 'You know the big chef?' referring to the television chef, 'He doesn't believe in stocks. Says the flavour is too strong for his food, so he boils up Rooster Booster for a while and that's how we made our stocks.'

Personally, at that moment, I was so into food (shall I say a bit of a purist?) I would have had him shot at dawn for such arrogance. To believe in the chemical over the substance was inconceivable. To get into good food guides using his powders was more evidence for me that those "food critics" knew little to nothing about food. To me, they were people without many skills who never had to pay for their meals. To charge top dollar for such subterfuge was immoral. This guy's ego was famous regarding his food ... but if a paying customer wanted the fish with vegetables instead of the salad advertised on the menu, they couldn't because his meals *'Weren't designed for that!'* Going against all that was hospitable – ego stomped on common sense. This may suggest that he liked to stand by his principles; but if he opens a tin and prefers that to something homemade (and still labels his food fresh and homemade), he doesn't have principles – he's just a tosser!

What amazed me was that he fooled some of the people

enough of the time (and we are talking the critics in Melbourne and Sydney) to still have his rather large fingers still in the restaurant game.

The chefs that I admired and had been fortunate enough to work under instilled in me a determination to make good, clear stocks. It was an art in itself. It took concentration and a certain reverence to the ingredients and resulting liquid. The subtle changes that go from water and meat and vegetables to a base for soups, sauces, stews are amazing – especially when you have to make 30 to 40 litre pots of the stuff. The whole kitchen (except desserts) relies on the quality of what you are making. If food on the plate is the body, then the stock has to be its soul.

I remember leaving a 20 litre bucket of chicken stock out overnight. Maybe it was the rush to get out after a long day made me forget. It was an accident, but to this arrogant chef, James (the other apprentice) and I had committed a major sin. I can still hear him saying: '*How many fucking birds died to make that pot of stock? And you treat them with such disrespect?*'

Disrespect was an unusual word for him to use because his understanding of respectful behaviour to me was starting the day with chanting: 'Rule number one: no poofters, rule number two: no poofters, and rule number three: consult rule number one.' He then would burst out laughing. The running joke became '*rule number one*' and that would make him laugh. He once accused me of going *"all girly"* every time a man walked into the kitchen and he said it revolted him.

The comment about chickens dying for the stock was one of the few intelligent things that he ever said and it left me thinking ... I'd just wasted the lives of about forty chickens. To see and smell what they had become in eight hours

– a rather putrid-smelling, bubbling liquid that had to be poured down the sink – was terrible. The aroma hung around for hours, even with the huge extractor fans on.

Normally so many gorgeous cooking smells just get sucked up and out, never to be smelt again, but if something has died, turned or just gone off that old feisty smell clings to the walls as if it is refuses to get pulled into the extractors. You can tip it all down the sink and wash it down with plenty of water, but that smell hangs – and it certainly did this day. So it's not something you want to leave out overnight, especially in summer. Maybe if you live in a cold climate or during winter – then you could probably get away with it. Ideally it's best to go into fridge cold but if it's still warm in the pot, on a cold night, it's probably okay to be left out and put in fridge in the morning.

* * *

Back at the hospital, I had awakened abruptly from another drug-induced sleep. It was about 7.30am when the Conscious Ones start clucking about with their trolleys. Memories of the sandwiches filled my head and a little smile spread across my face as I recalled savouring tiny mouthfuls of the soggy things. This was my fifth day of this seemingly meaningless torture, but I told myself it was for a reason: *They just don't know what it is about. They will get to it. If they keep me today – which I'm sure they are going to because I still am in pain and they're still unsure as to what is happening – something has to change. I'm not going to let them stuff me around anymore. I can't have this morphine. How can I tell them where it hurts when my head isn't even on the planet? Stupid drug! Stupid questions! Stupid doctors!*

It felt as if my life-force was physically slipping away

from me. I needed energy, needed to take my HIV drugs, which I'd had to stop because I wasn't allowed to eat. These medications needed to be taken with food.

I could feel I was going beyond my limit, whatever it was. Maybe it was the mental safety net where the pills gave me a certain quality of life. The HIV medication regime had been thrown into chaos along with my headspace. I knew that those two combined – bad headspace and sporadic pill taking – were going to get me into trouble. These doctors weren't even taking the ramifications of being off my meds into consideration.

A nurse came into the ward with a smile and said her good mornings then told me that the specialist would be coming in to see me at 8.30am. The specialist was the urologist who wanted to take my pancreas out. My response to the nurse was: 'I don't want to see anybody unless they are all here. They are torturing me and I refuse to let them anymore.'

'What do you mean "all of them"?'

'The urologist, the ward doctor, the Asian guy and the other one; they all want to take out different parts of me and they aren't going to unless they all settle on one thing! At a time! I'm not into psycho trips and they are doing it to me big time. I want to see them all at once.'

'Well! This is unusual. So we may need to reschedule the 8.30 to get them all in at one time ...' Away she went.

Go girl! I thought to myself. Mum and Dad rang and asked if they could get me anything.

'Mesclun.'

'What's that?'

'You know: the mixed baby lettuce you can buy with the different colours and flavours. A big handful.' About an hour later my parents came in with a freezer bag of lettuce which I started shoving into my mouth by the handful. I needed green and *alive*. It was urgent. Dad looked at me in a bizarre "how could you?" sort of way. It didn't satisfy hunger, but it did its bit to energize me.

As I shoved leaves into my mouth I turned to both of them and said: 'I'm sick of this. All the doctors are coming in at once and I'm going to give it to them.'

The nurse came in a bit later to ask how the pain was and if I needed anything.

I told her: 'Yes I'm in pain, but don't even think about giving me morphine because I ain't gonna be a blubbering idiot.'

Mum said: 'Gregory, don't give these people a hard time. They are here to help you, you know.' And with those parting words, kisses, hugs, and questions if I needed anything, they left.

As the gaggle of doctors (what is the collective noun for a group of doctors?) strutted into the ward for their examination, they all looked at me as if I was some troublemaker. The last one to arrive was the urologist. They all asked how the patient was. I told them that I had let them all do their torture treatments on me and asked why a simple colonic irrigation wasn't a preferred option, if I was so blocked, as opposed to four days of enemas. I told them how they were all responsible for stuffing up my medication regime and asked if they were aware that by doing this they were opening me up to any opportunistic infection. The front page of The Age newspaper this particular day was the Alfred Hospital's sterilising equipment in surgery unit had fucked up, which I just happened to have on my bed.

I asked them, speaking of my medication, if any of them had considered looking up the side effects. I went on ... well I was on a roll, and not being one to shy from the limelight.

'I know one of my medications' side effects causes kidney stones. That is Indinavir. Has anybody looked it up in their copy of MIMS?'

They all stood there looking at me slightly uncomfortably when the head nurse piped up: 'Colonic irrigation was an outdated thing from the 60's and we don't do treatments that can be harmful to our patients.'

My reply: 'And you allow what you call the kitchen to serve up Rooster Booster – that isn't even dissolved? And you also keep the drug companies alive by administering these so called non-harmful medications. Even though I have to eat to take my HIV drugs, you willingly put me on a nil-oral diet? A colonic irrigation lasts for about an hour and a half. You have kept me on these drugs for four and a half days. Personally, I don't see your rationale.' The head nurse didn't really like me. I just shot her down.

Apparently, you don't talk to doctors that way. But none of them had thought about my meds. They all stood back. It was obvious they hadn't looked into my pills because they all looked blank and collectively went to move away to discuss me out of earshot.

'Where are you going? I want to hear this!' I demanded.

They all looked so angry and, just to piss me off I'm sure, they spoke in medical jargon, with words that had more syllables than I could comprehend.

The ward doctor was the one who was sent to look up the MIMS dictionary. Five minutes later, they all collected around the bed to inform me that Indinavir causes stones that wouldn't be seen under the tests that I had been through. One of those nuclear-type tests was organised and off I was wheeled for the procedure.

I don't take well to rude people, and this urologist and anaesthetist certainly were. Admittedly, I was freaked out

START WITH YOUR OWN ONION

but finally something was going to happen. At 1.30pm I was wheeled into the surgery to have the most painful procedure of my life – one I hope I will ever have to endure again.

What does one do if they really want to tell someone they're a pompous turd, but they have just told you they are going to put a tube into you through the eye of your penis, through your bladder, to the tube that connects your kidney, and place a plastic stent in you "for your own good"? My reaction at that time was to keep my mouth shut.

The nurse, who had wheeled me down for the test, had had a confrontation with the two doctors over their treatment of me. She told me to make a complaint. I never did get around to that letter, but I feel I'm exorcising that demon now.

As I was being told of the procedure in the pre-op room and giving my details, I observed the uniformed man who was asking me my name and if I knew what was going on. He had a fabulous pair of biceps, with a relatively recent-looking tattoo on his left arm. I had to smile to myself. Even in all this, I was still checking out the trade! Naughty Gregory! They wheeled me in and for the next minute or so the anaesthetist explained what he was going to do and that I would be out soon. Mr. Tattoo said: 'Where's Coorabell?' Looking at my address. I replied that it overlooked Byron Bay 'Isn't that where that famous King's Beach is?'

All I remember was slurry 'Siiiissssstterrr' and I went into unconsciousness with a smile, imagining him on the beach with less of the uniform on ...

By four o'clock I was coming to and had been told that I could leave by six. Mum and Dad (always there) arrived at the ward by 5.30. I cried like a baby. IT WAS ALL OVER!!!!

As they wheeled me out of the hospital, amidst

farewells from the nurses, I couldn't wait to light a cigarette. In fact, my strongest desire was to do a "Patsy" and light five cigarettes at once. Being released from this jail (sorry, hospital) was one of the most exhilarating moments I can recall in my life. With those tentative steps towards the car, tears fell from my eyes. I was overjoyed.

How I craved for some real food. My mind saw visions of chocolate mousse, eye fillet steak, Tasmanian salmon, Nori rolls with delectable fillings ... But as we got home my stomach told me a boiled egg and some plain toast was probably the most appropriate thing for me to eat.

After a long, dead sleep in the spare room at Mum and Dad's, I knew the inevitable was about to happen. I hobbled into the toilet and stuffed my mouth with a face cloth and just sat. My brain said to let go. My other organs weren't forthcoming. They had been violated and they weren't about to obey anyone, including me.

Long deep breaths, I chanted in my head, but it was about half an hour before the flow started which seemed as if it would never end. I went almost to the point of losing consciousness. My soul seemed to roar through my body and travel up past Mars. In a strange way (through pain) I hit Nirvana. I had left my body sitting on the toilet seat and I was in the presence of God. There is no other way to explain what happened. My organs had finally let go. I was too weak to scream and my body took me somewhere I had never been.

When the flow subsided I had no energy to move for a good while. When I finally did, I felt I was about a hundred years old. I was so weak but so hungry. I needed to eat. Mum said she was going to the shops and asked if I needed anything. I looked in the fridge. She had some carrots and celery. I peered into the cupboard and saw bay leaves and onions. I told her to buy a free-range chicken, hokkien noodles and some necks.

Whilst she went down the street to the shops I prepared the vegetables. I peeled and chopped two medium carrots, cleaned and chopped two sticks of celery and two onions. I grabbed a few bay leaves and about ten peppercorns and put them in a large pot and waited for Mum to return.

She returned with the chicken which I took out of its bag, washed it and the necks in cold water, cut off its bum and placed them all in a pot with the vegetables and spices. I then filled the pot to about four centimetres over the chicken with water and put it on to boil.

After my second cup of tea the pot had come to the boil. I turned it down to simmer and left it for an hour or so. At this stage it was time to put on some Aretha Franklin and do a major chill. The aroma of chicken stock cooking is a wonderful, homelike smell; old-fashioned in a way, majorly comforting. I like to describe it as a grandma smell.

With the noodles, I opened the packet, put them into a large bowl, poured boiling water over them, then let them sit for a few minutes, drained them in a colander and divided them into the serving bowls.

I removed the chicken from the stock and cut the two legs up roughly. I discarded the skin and bones, then added the flesh to the bowls. I then checked the flavour of the stock added salt to taste. This I poured over the noodles and chicken with some of the stock vegetables and I added some fish sauce and tamari (or soy sauce), a good squeeze of lemon juice and a teaspoon of sesame oil per bowl.

My stomach grumbled as the food went down. I ended up having three bowls and I knew I was back on Earth with a full, content stomach.

The ordeal over – until the removal of the stent, but that

was definitely far from my mind and a thought for another day.

* * *

Preparing a Bird for Cooking

My Liberian sister Augustina says that you should always prepare a fresh bird by squeezing fresh lime or lemon juice over it then rub maybe a couple of teaspoons of salt over it. Leave this for a few minutes then wash it completely. This is to clean the chicken and destroy bacteria that could have spilt on the chicken when it was processed or during handling.

My dear friend Clement, who is Malaysian by birth and was taught how to cook by his mother, says the salt and juice is rubbed all over the chicken as it makes the skin silkier.

My dear friend Joanne, a brilliant chef, restaurateur and food business owner, has said that it isn't necessary in Australia with Australian standards.

I say when I buy a new shirt, towel, sheets I generally give them a wash before I put them on. So if you're going to put it in your mouth I don't mind giving a bird a wash. I do know I have used vinegar when I have been out of lemons or limes. It doesn't hurt it.

* * *

Clement's Hainan Method

- Wash the chicken then rub salt all over it for a few minutes. This is to give the finished product a certain look

START WITH YOUR OWN ONION

- It's not necessary to wash it again, but just be aware of how much salt you have used
- If you have used a lot then you could wash it off. Salt reduces the pimply look, keeping the skin smooth
- Cut off excess fat, Popes nose and pull off loose feathers
- Don't discard the fat as that can be chopped up finely and used in the rice pilaf instead of using oil
- Add a good knob of garlic and a thumb sized piece of ginger that have been given a good squash or rough chop to a pot of chicken stock
- Bring that just to the boil. Not a lot of movement is needed
- Place 2 spring onions cut in thirds into the cavity of the chook then breast down place the chook in the stock and bring up to a simmer
- Turn off the heat and let sit for ½ to ¾ of an hour
- Turn the chicken over on its back and bring up to a simmer again
- Repeat the process.

* * *

Beef Stock and Game Stocks

If you don't have the best ventilation in your home, or don't have time for these longer cooking stocks, then it might be best to buy them. Ventilation problems can be overcome to a degree by roasting bones on a BBQ and cooking the stock on the side burner if it has one. Just be aware: roasting beef or game bones then cooking them for several hours can leave a strong, fatty sort of smell. The methods are pretty much all the same:

- Roast an amount of bones and veggies that you have a pot big enough for
- Add to a pot of cooked bones, mirepoix (vegies), water with some bay leaves and peppercorns and cook slowly for at least 3 to 4 hours
- It should only be brought to a boil and then turned down to simmer on a very low heat
- It's then strained and left to sit
- To get rid of the oil and fat that floats on top lightly drag paper towel across the top of the stock also it can be left till it goes cold and the fat can be lifted off in one go.

* * *

Fish Stock

For fish stock, fish heads are great. One decent sized (around 800gms) schnapper head will make enough stock for soup for about eight people. Get them scaled if you're buying them, or if you caught them scale them yourself. It's always good to give them a wash in cold water.

- To about 800gms or more of fish bones add 1 large carrot, 2 chopped brown onions, 2 sticks of celery, 2 or 3 bay leaf and pepper corns.
- If you choose you can add sprigs of fennel, dill or part of a fennel bulb or a teaspoon of fennel seeds or even a splash of Pernod at the end.
- Cover the bones and vegies in water and bring it to a boil. As soon as it's started to bubble, turn

the heat down to a simmer and cook for about ½ hour.
- A great soup is made from schnapper head this way. There is a great amount of flesh in the cheeks. Once it's cooked take the head out of the stock and let cool.
- Carefully peel back the skin and collect the flesh from the head. This can be served in a similar way to Shanes' Hainan Chicken.

* * *

Vegetable Stock

A lot of the classically trained chefs I worked with never put too much effort in a vegetable stock.

Method 1:

Often they were the scraps, trimmings and peel from everywhere else. It was never an exact science at all. It was treated with a bit of contempt. For most of them it was just scraps of whatever vegetable matter was available all put in a pot and boiled and at the end Worchester sauce was added.

Method 2:

The pot was given all the scraps of just about any vegetable then water (including water that had been used to steam or blanche vegetables) added, and it was boiled for a while then strained. It never was a brilliant thing. Even made worse one time when I followed the rule to the letter and didn't think about the effect that beetroot trimmings would add to the stock. Ultimately the beetroot gave it a rather interesting colour possibly not a desired one though.

Method 3 (my version):

- After thinking what I need the stock for, generally I use water!
- You can use a few onions, carrots and a stick of celery or two in some water (you can roast the veggies first if you like) and cook the stock for a few hours. This is pretty time consuming
- If I'm making a vegetarian soup or stew, I tend to skip the stock making and just add those vegetables to the soup or stew I'm making. I have found when making a sauce or soup where a vegetable stock is needed I use water and add those vegetables onions, carrot celery that would be used for the stock to the recipe being used. For instance, a cauliflower soup I would be sweating off a mirepoix of carrot, onion, celery and adding the cauliflower and water and any other ingredients desired
- I have also found possibly the most flavoursome vegetable stock is the water used when pressure cooking chick peas. It has a real nutty, delicious flavour that shouldn't be thrown out, but used wherever a stock is needed.

* * *

Miso Soup

The closest thing to instant I know is a good dessertspoon of miso paste in a cup of boiling water. You have a satisfying drink that is soothing and calmative on a stomach. It's an easy meal to steam some veggies and rice with a cup of miso.

* * *

My Asian-Inspired Broth

2 onions
1 bunch coriander – roots well-washed
2 red chillies
1 good sized knobs of ginger
2 sticks of lemon grass
6 cardamom pods
6 cloves garlic
2 limes leaves
1 star anise

Stock of choice – chicken, beef, vegetable, fish or miso can be used.

If you're making a vegetarian broth as the base you could add onion some carrot and celery. The pleasure of this recipe is you can use as much or as little of most ingredients as you like. If you don't like chilli then don't use it. If you do like it hot, then use more. Simple!

- Sweat onions (I like to get these well-cooked till caramelised)
- Add garlic, ginger, chillies, lemon grass, then spices
- Then to the pot add the desired stock
- Let this cook for ½ hour or so letting the

flavours blend
- Take off heat. Now it can be strained and then finished off
- Season the soup with soy, fish sauce and lemon/lime juice
- Serve with steamed rice, tofu, by itself, with dumplings, noodles or vegetables.

* * *

Prawn or Shellfish Stock

The job of peeling prawns (or any crustacean that's edible) is never the best fun. After you peel them to avoid stinky fingers, wash your fingers in lemon juice, then cold, soapy water. Next warm soapy water this will tend to get rid of the smell. I was told that if you washed your hands straight away in hot water the smell can seep into your skin. I make prawn stock from the shells and heads if I have fresh or cooked.

- After peeling, instead of discarding the shells and heads, put them all into a pot cover with water add a mirepoix consisting of onion, carrot, celery and bay leaf. I often put a clove or two of garlic in for good measure
- Same process as the fish stock it doesn't need a lot of cooking so bring it to a boil then turn it down and let simmer for about half an hour
- Strain and it can be frozen for another day
- This stock is best used as a basis for a soup, risotto, seafood stew or a pasta sauce
- My favourite thing to do with this shellfish stock is the bisque recipe later on.

TWO
PLAYING WITH METHODS

When you have watched someone in absolute pain, and when that person has been offered everything to dull the pain and nothing works ... would you be willing to try anything? If that person was your greatest love or child, parent or friend what would you do? When you accept the inevitable: that your loved one is going to die, and the only thing you can do is watch whilst doctors and medical people try to help to alleviate pain what would you do?

* * *

1995

Max never liked morphine even though he had to use it. He was such an articulate man but when he went to speak on the drug his brain would work but his mouth wouldn't. It was as if on top of everything else, his dignity was being attacked. This incredibly emotional experience became a bit complicated when words would fall out of his mouth, then he would get a pained expression on his face which meant what he had said was not what he actually wanted to say.

Trying to decipher what his intent was became a little game. I tended to try and distract him with anything that came to mind. He did appreciate my taste in music, so the ultimate distraction was Aretha or Nina Simone or even Millie Jackson. I would put on a screaming black Shelia or at the other end of the scale some classical music, whatever the situation could handle to help alleviate his mood.

I never appreciated the ability to speak until I saw my dear friend unable to. It was a similar experience to me not appreciating the ability to urinate until I struggled to after the kidney stones. Max would have good days where he wouldn't take the dose of morphine and he would say to me: 'Now about last Thursday when we were talking about ...' He would remember and say the sentence that his brain and mouth couldn't get out on that particular Thursday. These, admittedly, were rare moments.

My dear friend Max faded away before my eyes in what now seems like a horrible nightmare. He had skin cancers, ulcers the size of golf balls in his oesophagus and lower intestines, and a myriad of other diseases that were attacking his whole system. His tongue needed to be coated in a lubricant (which tasted foul) because he had stopped salivating. His system hovered near to collapse for close to six months. Anti-nausea pills and painkillers, combined with marijuana, eased the situation.

A routine was set. After waking up, Max would venture out of his bedroom and lie on his couch. On a glass table, in the morning sun, was a crystal vase three quarters filled with water. In that was a plastic drink container with the bottom cut out and a cone positioned in the lid of the drink container. The single most glamorous bucket bong that you could imagine, because as you inhaled and it went down it was positioned so the morning sun created millions of prisms. Only a true creative Queen could be so theatrical.

Max and I were introduced to each other by a mutual friend, Wayne. We had been diagnosed at a similar time. Unfortunately, Max was well and truly into the disease and was ravaged by the experience. He had two large indents in his face where cancers had been removed even before his diagnosis. He was treated for cancer but not given a HIV test because at that time they operated a connection to this particular type of cancer and HIV possibly wasn't established (or some doctor was really lazy).

He had large Kaposi sarcoma on his body that eventually grew over his face. We had both been invited to a mutual friend's place for lunch. We both lived in Suffolk Park and, me not having a car at the time, Wayne organized for Max to give me a lift.

I am always impressed when you meet someone for the first time and within minutes they pull out a joint. We laughed all the way to Wayne's place about fifteen minutes away, and all that afternoon.

Max was one of those few genuine people that I've met in life, where an instant rapport was a long-lasting one. Although I only knew him in this life for about 18 months, his smile and laugh will be with me always.

I started to go around to Max's place during the day to help him out. We became firm friends. I'd noticed that he had a fan-forced oven in the kitchen. I got very excited. I told him that I had a chocolate cake recipe that needed that style of oven and asked if I could use it.

We loved chocolate, good coffee, black-American female soul, blues, gospel singers, and good food. Because of our recent diagnoses, we were going through similar emotions. We ended up laughing at them. It's amazing how many tasteless death jokes you can make when you're dealing with your mortality. None of which I'm going to repeat.

On my 28th birthday I arrived at Max's to do some housework and to check up on him. He had been very weak and in bed for a few days. I opened the door to find him sitting at his baby grand piano and he played "Happy Birthday" to me with lots of flourishes and hand movements. It was one of the best gifts I have ever been given. For a moment I saw a happy, well, and active man – relishing playing the piano and giving a gift that he knew I would love. At the end I needed to help him to a better chair. I was a bit of a mess needing tissues – nose dribbling – but he laughed and said: 'Happy Birthday, love!'

Marijuana is an appetite stimulant. Most HIV drugs I had been on at this time were appetite suppressants. If they weren't directly suppressants, it was all the vomiting that went on with the drugs that destroyed my appetite. If I lost my breakfast and morning medication, doctors told me that I should have some more breakfast and take my pills again. I don't know anybody who achieved this successfully without the help of the herb. If I had lost my breakfast a small joint was the way to go to settle the stomach and mind to be able to repeat the process.

Max had it down pat. He had two cones before breakfast to help start being hungry and then, as they kicked in, painkillers to ease the pain of the ulcers. This was my cue; I made sure breakfast was as big as possible. It had to be timed really well as a simple trip to the loo could throw the whole pain management out of kilter. If it didn't cause grief before it hit his stomach then it was after it left his stomach and on to the intestines that it did. So timing was every-

START WITH YOUR OWN ONION

thing, because he didn't want to get too out of it. He wanted to be able to do things that were still within his grasp. Maybe not a walk on the beach, but certainly he wanted to sit on the beach. He found that with a lot of the painkillers that he just became a zombie.

Max loved his crystal vase bucket bong. When the doctors say: *'Whatever makes the patient comfortable.'* You get to a point where you are willing to try anything to help ease pain. The vase bong was the ultimate. And then there were the cookies.

At one of the local markets on the Northern Rivers was a wonderful character who sold fabulous marijuana cake. Everybody was aware of this lady, and she never let anyone down. It was at this time when I started to experiment with the idea of eating the beautiful herb.

After several attempts I have found that to cook the leaf in butter in a crock-pot is the go. If a crock-pot wasn't available then cooking it on the stove over a very low heat.

I've left the butter to stew in the crock for about three or four hours, or on the stove at least half an hour to an hour. I have found that some people's methods are to put some water in the stove pot to stop it from catching.

Another friend of mine got scientific about the process and would blanche the leaf or head then wrap it in a tea towel and leave to sit overnight before cooking, which he believed broke down the THC molecules and more goodness was released. This does work well, but all the water must be cooked out before you use the butter.

Another method for end result is to strain the butter and use that. I think that has enormous waste potential. What I do is to puree the whole lot, butter and herb when it's cool puree in a food processor. Once it's a fine paste, and put into a container to solidify it then can be used in most biscuit or cake mixtures. It should be a fabulous dark black green paste.

My favourite recipe and simplest is based on a sable biscuit. The trick with most butter, sugar, flour biscuit recipes is not to over-whip the butter and sugar. Too much beating at this stage will make a crumbly biscuit that is lovely and light but will not hold. The whipping incorporates air which makes it fluffy but also makes it very hard to handle. This mix can be used as a flan or tart base but if it's too airy it won't hold well as a base!

* * *

Base Recipe Sable Biscuits

(Great base for sweet tarts and flans)
350gm butter
150gm icing sugar
500gm flour
I generally use ¾ my herb butter and ¼ normal butter

- In a mix master (if you're feeling strong this can easily be done by hand) lightly beat the butter and sugar, then add flour till it combines
- At this stage I think of the end result. The marijuana has a strong flavour, so I like to chop up a block of chocolate or a hand full of dried fruit and add to the mixture
- Get a handful of dough and roll into tubes.
- Slice them and place them evenly apart on a lined baking tray
- Bake for about 20 minutes until golden brown and firm to the touch.

When you eat, always have half or a quarter of a cookie and give yourself an hour at least before you start downing more because by then you will know how strong they are.

If you had a male plant that you were growing in the back yard and you've used this for your butter, then that's usually not going to be as strong as if you've used an ounce of heads from a female plant. Personally, I have always preferred to cook the leaf because it is unpleasant to smoke. Therefore my recipe above is based on using leaf.

I get approximately 30 to 32 biscuits out of each batch from the above recipe. If you have used an ounce of strong stuff then just beware – decrease the amount of herb butter and balance with normal butter you put in the dough.

This recipe is for something that I believe some people can have allergic reactions to just the same as having an allergic reaction to broccoli, strawberries or peanuts. If you believe that you may have a reaction to it then don't do it.

My opinion of people who believe that marijuana should be banned is low. I do believe every house on the planet should have its own crop. Alas! The people that make painkillers would go out of business. The generation that were teenagers during the 1960's that are closer now to their sixties, were a great disappointment. The generation that lived through The Doors, Janis Joplin, The Rolling Stones, Jimi Hendrix, Joe Cocker and even The Beatles couldn't get it together to have pot legalized by the time that they retire, when they really need it. I don't just blame the sixties generation. Each and every generation has failed in its ability to deal effectively with people dying with dignity.

* * *

It's always good to have a selection of normal biscuits that you can have when the munchies kick in! This is an old classic CWA recipe that in recent years has come back as an uber-expensive morsel. It's pretty simple and easy.

* * *

Almond Bread

    4 egg whites (120ml)
    4oz sugar (125gm)
    4oz flour (125gm)
    4oz almonds (skins on) these can be replaced with any nuts but they do need to have the skin on as the skin sticks to the mixture and this stops the nut from falling through when slicing the loaf. Nuts like pecans, walnuts, almonds, hazelnuts etc are perfect. If you try Macadamias or even peanuts they need to be chopped smaller but still they can have a tendency to fall out.

- Whip whites till peaking which means they have literally tripled in volume (or more) and they are stiff. This should take just a few minutes
- Slowly start to add sugar
- When they are stiff and the sugar is well combined with a rubber spatula or large spoon fold in the flour. This means pour half the flour on top of the mixture starting from the centre dive the spatula into the centre and drag the contents up the side of the bowl. Once started keep going making sure the flour is getting incorporated then add the second half and keep

going. Folding in the flour needs a certain amount of speed
- Now fold through the nuts
- Pour into a loaf tin lined with baking paper
- Bake in a loaf tin in a moderate oven (180C) for about ¾ hour to an hour. When it's ready it will be firm to the touch
- Take out of the oven and cool on a rack. If you don't have a rack then a chopping board but when it's cooling give it an occasional turn to stop it from getting soggy on one surface
- When cool, wrap in a clean tea towel and leave in a cool spot till the next day (a good 24 hours later)
- Slice the loaf. Place slices on a baking tray and re-bake slices in a slow oven (130c) up to half an hour till lightly golden, cool on a rack
- For something a bit fancy take half the mixture, (after adding the nuts) and fold a tablespoon of cocoa through this half. Then when the mixes are put together lightly swirl them and then proceed with baking.

* * *

Meringues

250ml egg whites (approx 8 eggs)
250gm castor sugar
200gm icing sugar
25gm corn flour

- This is the same process as the almond bread
- Mix the corn flour with the icing sugar

- In a mix master whip whites slowly adding sugars and cornflour
- Turn machine onto high and whip till firm the mixture is good and stiff. This should take about 4-5 minutes
- If you want to make a nut meringue a few tablespoons of a nut meal hazelnut, macadamia, cashew, walnut etc can be folded through at this stage
- When mixture is ready it should pipe out nicely. If it's sloppy you haven't beaten it enough
- Pipe onto trays or scoop onto trays depending on what you desire your end result to be
- Bake in a slow oven (100C) for a few hours till firm
- Turn off oven and these can stay in the oven overnight.

* * *

Anzac Biscuits

130gm butter (unsalted butter is better to use for sweet biscuits)
1 tablespoon of golden syrup
1 cup plain flour
Pinch salt
1 cup coconut
1 cup sugar
1 cup rolled oats
2 teaspoons of bi carb soda
2 tablespoons boiling water

- Melt the butter, golden syrup, and water together and add bi carb soda then all the dry ingredients
- Scoop or roll small drops about a heaped teaspoon size onto a tray lined with baking paper
- Bake for about 20 minute's in a moderate oven
- Depending if you like chewy or hard: bake the cookies for a bit shorter time for chewy or a bit longer for hard
- Place them on a baking rack to cool.

* * *

Biscotti

The almonds used in this recipe can be substituted for any other nut. What you need is a third of ground nuts (meal) and two thirds chopped or slivered or any other variation.

4 oz (125gm) of blanched almonds
2 ½ cups of plain flour
¾ cup of caster sugar
3 eggs
Salt
1 teaspoon of baking soda
3 oz (approx 90gm) of semi-sweet chocolate chopped into small chunks
1 extra-large egg white

- Toast the almonds when cool grind a third, chop the rest (roughly)

- Pour all the dry ingredients into a bowl, mix well, forming a well in the centre
- Add eggs (except the one white) and combine to dough
- Once all combined let it rest for ¼ to ½ hour
- Roll into tubes and place each tube on a baking sheet lined with baking paper
- Bake at 180C (375F) for 20 minutes
- Remove tray from the oven and when the tubes are still warm cut into diagonal shapes and place them back on the tray cut side down
- Lower oven temperature to 100C (225F) and re-bake for 30 minutes.

* * *

Brandy Snaps

These can be a bit of a pain but for a special occasion they are ok and they are at the moment sort of retro and in fashion! I put the three amounts here in columns because it just reminds me of different occasions where volumes become important. The smallest batch will do about 20 tubes.

350gm flour | 175gm flour | 90gm flour
350gm butter | 175gm butter | 90gm butter
375gm golden syrup | 180gm GS | 90gm GS
850gm icing sugar | 425gm IS | 210gm IS

* * *

Brandy Snap Baskets
170gm golden syrup

340gm castor sugar
170gm butter
9gm ground ginger
140gm plain flour
Zest of a lemon

Brandy snaps and baskets have the same method of combining ingredients, can be the same recipe and have a similar result. They are essentially different shapes. With the combination of orange, lime, lemon, any citrus zest or some interesting spice the end result can be a real marriage of flavours.

- The method to both recipes is to melt the butter and golden syrup in a pot on the stove
- Once melted, it shouldn't be hot, just liquid; add the spices and zest, if any desired and then the flour
- Combine well and set aside, cover with a cloth in a bowl till cool.

For a tube snap to be filled with cream:

- Place small teaspoon size of dough on the baking sheet. The dough will spread a lot so bake one at first and see how far it spreads. The idea is you don't want them to bake together (when hot they can be cut if they have run together)
- Bake in a moderate oven for about 10 minutes

- Give the biscuit a minute or two when out of the oven then when still warm, with a spatula lift it off the tray and then with your hands roll it around the handle of a wooden spoon or any tube you have (no pun intended on that one). You have to be quick if you have put ten on a tray – it helps to have asbestos fingers! Preferably using a wide head spatula to scrape them off the tray you need to be quick and have a few wooden spoons
- Leave to cool on the handles of the wooden spoons then slide off.

The method for the basket shape:

- The method for the brandy snap basket differs only at the after pulling out of the oven stage
- The baskets are easier in that when out of the oven, they can be flipped onto an upended glass, cup or a dariole mould; something that can give it a flat surface and sides
- Let it hang down the sides till cool
- These can last a few days in a airtight container. They could last longer as long as really airtight.

* * *

Cornets

These are a similar thing to the brandy snap in that they are made as a thin biscuit or a biscuit to hold a dessert in. I've cut out shapes on an ice cream container lid and used that as a mould to get desired shapes. I've made baskets and biscuits called "Cats Tongue" all sorts of shapes including butterflies folded over the wooden spoon handle to get the fold in the wings. A bit of effort can be a great end result.

8oz (250gms) butter
8oz sugar
8 egg whites
8oz plain flour

- Cream butter and sugar. This means that in a mix master you put the paddle shaped implement into the machine and beat the butter and sugar together till they turn white-ish
- On a low speed add the egg whites slowly, then the flour
- Onto a baking tray lined with baking paper shape onto tray. They only need to be a few millimetres thick. They shouldn't spread much if they are thin
- Bake till brown on 150C (300F) should take about 10 minutes
- When they are the desired colour take out and curl to desired shape as in a cone or similar to brandy snap baskets. They won't bend as much as the brandy snaps, so just beware it has limitations.

* * *

Crostolli

Crostolli is a bit of a favourite but I don't seem to have it very often. I was going to put a few different versions of a recipe down as I have made them all but I find Marcella Hazan's recipe is the best. I have used vegetable fat and butter but for me the end result never got the crisp that lard gets. It's not a delicate thing to eat if its coated in icing or fine confectioner's sugar, but that's half the fun.

* * *

Marcella Hazan – Chiacchiere Della Nonna – Sweet Pastry Fritters

(*what I'd call Crostolli*)
200gm plain flour
60gm lard for the dough and at least 300gm for frying
1 tablespoon sugar
1 egg
2 tablespoons of white wine
1 teaspoon of salt
Icing sugar to dust

- Rub with your hands the 60gm of softened lard into the flour that already has the tablespoon of sugar and salt mixed through
- Now add the egg white
- Knead until the dough is nice and smooth
- Cover with plastic wrap and let it rest for 15 minutes
- Roll and cut into 3mm thick 12cm long bow shapes
- Fry in 1 inch deep of lard in a frypan or pot until light brown and crisp. Be careful not to get the fat too hot keep it around 180C
- When finished cooking lift onto a paper towel

to let drain then roll in a bowl of icing sugar or fine castor sugar whilst still warm.

* * *

Dutch Biscuits

I'm not sure as to why these are called Dutch but they are another simple shortbread type biscuit that with a bit of creativity some cocoa or some other colour can get some great two toned biscuits.

300gm flour
   1 ½ teaspoons baking powder
   125gm sugar icing
   Vanilla essence/rum essence
   4 tablespoons milk
   100gm soft butter

- Combine all the ingredients together till it's a fine smooth dough
- Split the mixture in half
- To one half add 2 tablespoons of cocoa
- Mix through
- Add dark and white together either by just combining and rolling into tubes or for a spiral effect roll out one to a rectangle then the other place one on top of the other and then roll them up tightly
- Let the tubes firm up in the fridge then slice and onto a baking tray lined with baking paper bake 180C (350F) for about 10 minutes

- When they are a golden colour take them out and place them on a wire (baking) rack.

*** * * ***

Gingerbread
125gm butter
½ cup brown sugar
1 egg yolk
2 ½ cups flour
1 teaspoon bicarb soda
3 teaspoon ground ginger
½ teaspoon cinnamon
½ teaspoon cardamom
½ teaspoon cloves
2 ½ tablespoons golden syrup

- Cream butter and sugar till combined well. It doesn't have to be ultra-whipped
- Add yolks and combine well then slowly add the flour, bicarb and spices. The dry ingredients can be sifted together first
- Wrap in a tea towel or in plastic wrap and let the dough rest for at least ½ hour
- Knead the dough lightly and then roll onto a floured bench or between layers of plastic wrap to about 3mm
- If you want gingerbread men then you cut them out or for whatever shape desired lay biscuits onto a lined baking sheet for 180C for 10 minutes
- A double mixture does a decent-sized gingerbread house and 'outhouse':

START WITH YOUR OWN ONION

- 1 x 26cm round base
- 2 x 20cm wide x 14cm high wall front and back of house
- 2 x 22cm wide x 10 high roof (peaked front and back)
- 2 x 12cm wide x up to 14cm high side walls. The side walls are a 5 sided shape fitting the slanted or 'A' framed roof.
- Just enough to make an outdoor dunny for Santa to have a pit stop on!

* * *

Royal Icing

1 lb (500gm) of icing sugar
3 egg whites
¼ teaspoon cream of tartar

- Whip the whites and start adding the dry ingredients
- Make sure the meringue is very stiff. This is the "glue" to build the house
- You need to act relatively fast so make sure you have all your decorations on hand to build the house
- A few pairs of hands works really fun. For a few Christmas's I did enjoy getting all the kids involved they are great memories

Note: if you try to make this on a really humid Christmas Day take my advice: DON'T!! I have funny memories of trying to keep the bloody gingerbread house together with Majella and Finn's hands keeping up the walls. Unfortunately the humidity just seemed to work against the icing. If it's typical summer in Australia and very humid try making at night a few days before if it's better weather.

* * *

Haakons
    300gm flour
    250gm butter
    100gm icing sugar
    1 egg yolk
    60gm almond meal
    100gm coffee crystals
    50gm chopped hazelnuts

- Combine butter, sugar, flour and meal following the same principle as the previous biscuits. Remember not to over whip the butter and sugar
- When combined roll into tubes and glaze with yolk and roll in crystals and hazelnut
- Put into fridge to let firm up
- Cut and place onto baking paper and bake for about 10 minutes on 180C
- When golden take out of oven and slide onto a wire rack to cool.

* * *

Melting Moments
Nana Young made the best Melting Moments and

START WITH YOUR OWN ONION

Mum loves a cup of tea and some of these! I know there is a sense of nostalgia for her in every mouthful.

¼ lb butter
    2 tablespoon icing sugar
    1 teaspoon of lemon zest
    1 cup cornflour
    1 cup SR flour

- Lightly beat butter and sugar
- Add zest and flours
- Roll into balls and press onto the tray
- Fork an impression to squash the balls into a flatter shape (dip fork into flour before making impressing to prevent it from sticking)
- Bake (180C) until firm about 10 minutes, but try not to colour the biscuit too much
- Cool on wire racks
- Sandwich together with icing recipe

* * *

Lemon Filling (optional)
    1 tablespoon butter
    4 tablespoon icing
    1 teaspoon lemon zest
    1 dessert spoon of sweetened condensed milk

- Combine soft butter with rest of ingredients

* * *

GREGORY KELLY

Yo-Yos
    6oz butter
    6oz SR flour
    2oz castor sugar
    2oz custard flour

Now I'm hoping you have picked up on the method it's relatively the same as before:

- Cream butter and sugar add flours
- Bake in a moderate oven till golden brown.

* * *

Shortbread
One thing that has always puzzled me about this traditional recipe is the inclusion of rice flour in the dough. Scotland is not really a place I thought rice would be grown in and have always been curious where that came from.

250gms butter
    2 tablespoons of ground rice or rice flour
    1/3 cup icing sugar
    2 cups of plain flour

- As above don't over beat the butter and sugar
- Shape as desired and bake till golden brown.

* * *

Orange Biscuits

250gm butter
Zest of one orange
350gm flour
200gm sugar
Pinch salt

- Cream butter and sugar then add zest, flour and salt
- These can be rolled into balls and sliced in half, baked and later sandwiched with some dark chocolate. However you shape them they are good with chocolate
- Bake moderate oven 15 minutes.

* * *

Chocolate Fudge Cookies
200gm dark chocolate
180gm unsalted butter
¼ cup glace ginger
2/3 cup caster sugar
3 large eggs
2 teaspoons vanilla
1 ½ cups flour
3 tablespoons of cocoa
½ teaspoon salt
½ teaspoon baking powder
1 cup icing

- Melt chocolate and butter together leave till a bit cool then add the eggs
- Followed by all the dry ingredients, except icing sugar

- Roll into ball shapes about half the size of a golf ball and roll in the icing sugar
- When placing on lined baking sheet push down slightly don't over crowd your baking tray as they do spread
- Keep the rest of the rolled balls in the fridge till needed to be baked
- These give a groovy effect when baked a sort of mottled cracked effect
- Bake for 12 minutes in a moderate oven cool on racks
- If you line the tray with several pieces of brown paper or butchers paper then the baking paper to cook the biscuits, it reduces direct heat and helps biscuits from over-cooking.

***

Ciambella (one) Ciambelle (two) (Phonetic Jump Ella)

These are an Italian Easter biscuit but I would call them more like a bun rolled into decent sized doughnut shapes that get painted with egg white sprinkled with sugar then baked. A painted egg (or chocolate egg) is then placed in the hole after baking and cooling. This was from Ivana, our pasta maker at the Queenscliff Hotel. Something her mother had taught her and I'm sure her mother's mother had taught her. The recipe in the left column is the one she gave to me. I've halved it in the right column as it is a big mixture.

Just under 1lb of butter | 225gm butter
About 300gm sugar | 150gm sugar

START WITH YOUR OWN ONION

1 cup pernod | ½ cup pernod
6 eggs (separate 1 egg white) | 3 eggs (separate 1)
1 teaspoon salt | ½ teaspoon salt
1 cup milk | ½ cup milk
1200gm SR flour | 600gm SR flour
Lemon zest | Lemon zest
Extra castor sugar for decorating

- Combine all together following the standard method of creaming butter with the sugar
- Adding salt, eggs and some of the flour, the liquids then the rest of the flour
- When combined roll into tubes and then add shape like a small doughnut making sure there is enough central space to place an egg
- Paint with egg white and sprinkle with the extra caster sugar
- Bake in a moderate oven till firm to touch and are lightly golden about 15-20 minutes.

* * *

Almond Numbers

Now again I've put 3 columns here and just multiplied the volumes. So if you are making for a friend or family follow the 3 egg, 180gm castor, 125gm almond and 110 butter recipe. Its only 4 ingredients so it's very easy. These are an interesting biscuit that can be a bit 'eggy' in flavour, so use small eggs. I like them but I can see why others wouldn't rave about them. They are a flat biscuit and require a bit of double baking.

1 dozen eggs | 6 eggs | 3 eggs

750gm castor sugar | 375gm CS | 180gm CS
500gm almond meal | 250gm AM | 125gm AM
450gm butter | 225gm butter | 110gm butter

- Ingredients are put together and drop teaspoon sized drops on a tray.
- They spread out so not too many on the tray
- About 7 or 8 minutes in a moderate (180°C) oven, bring the tray out.
- With a spatula turn them over and give them another 4 or 5 minutes
- Cool on a wire rack.

* * *

Almond Number 2 (no-bake)

This recipe really only has three ingredients icing sugar, almond meal and rose water. The almond meal can be any other nut meal and the rose water can be substituted for orange blossom water, pomegranate syrup or even a bit of sugar syrup and a blast of a liquor. So for example:

4 tablespoons almond meal
4 tablespoons icing sugar
About a tablespoon rose water

- Mix together icing sugar and almond meal and add small amounts of rose water until it forms a mix
- Roll into balls and roll in more icing sugar
- I store in the fridge
- Can be dipped in chocolate for a bit more luxury.

* * *

Gluten Free Peanut Numbers

400gm can of condensed milk

½ cup crunchy peanut butter (I've used cashew and hazelnut butters)

2 cups shredded coconut

1 ½ - 2 cups of nuts and seeds any variety (except salted but if this is all you have lightly wash and dry in a tea towel before use)

- Mix all ingredients together roll into balls and put on a baking tray lined with baking paper
- Bake in moderate oven for 8 minutes or lightly browned
- Cool on wire rack (this recipe makes about 35)

* * *

Susie's Vegan Numbers

1 ripe banana, mashed

1 cup oats

1 tablespoon coconut or Rapadura sugar

1 tablespoon cacao or cocoa

1 tablespoon shredded coconut

100gms of good vegan chocolate chopped up

A dash of vanilla essence

½ teaspoon cinnamon

- Mix and spoon onto parchment. Drop onto tray.
- Bake at 190C for 15 minutes
- Cool on parchment on rack.

THREE
FORMATIONS FOR A METHOD

The day I was diagnosed, over 27 years ago now, I recall eating quite a bit of chocolate.

I was really pissed off at the receptionist at the doctor's clinic. I had many tests over the years, the results of which took two weeks to come back.

It was not uncommon to get a false positive test, and you would have to go back for another test. This had happened twice to me. One test came back positive the next said I wasn't. It was quite emotional.

This time the Doctor had said to me that the receptionist, Anita, had left my blood on the counter and forgot to do whatever they do to it, so it had gone "off". I walked out of his office at the end of this visit and abused Anita for being so careless with *my* blood.

So I had to have another blood test which required another two weeks of waiting. When my results returned the doctor told me that the tests had both come back positive. I remember saying: *'Both tests?'*

To which the doctor replied: 'Well what I said last time wasn't exactly correct. The results needed to be verified, because you've had false positive tests. So we repeat the test to make sure there isn't a mistake.'

'You mean I went out and verbally abused Anita for being slack – and she wasn't slack, you were just gutless?'

'Well I wouldn't say gutless. I didn't want to alarm you if the test had been wrong.'

'I virtually ripped the shit out of a woman who I was told had been reckless with my blood and now you tell me she wasn't? You just didn't want to tell me the truth. Doctor, you are a prick!'

I was concerned that I'd been really horrible to this woman, and that I'd made a huge performance. I told everybody I knew how Anita had fucked up when it wasn't her fuck-up at all!

All of Byron's groovy crew went to this guy because he was into Chinese medicine as well as Western medicine. It helped to be able to talk to a younger man who was hip to the world. All the dance crew went to him when they were coming down off bad eccies or trips or whatever they had taken at the last party – Doctor would fix them up. Actually, I found that you could spend more time talking to Doctor about the last party he'd been to than whatever your complaint was. Sometimes I would go to see him and end up forgetting to ask him what I was there for. That used to shit me.

One time, I had to ride back to the surgery about eight kilometres because I forgot to get a prescription – having got carried away talking about the last "Tropical Fruits" party.

On the day of my diagnosis, after Doctor had said all that needed to be said. I walked out to face Anita. I hadn't really heard anything he'd said after the diagnosis. The only thing I was conscious of was how horribly rude I had been to her – and that, in case I did kick it tomorrow, I needed to apologise to her immediately.

I looked at Anita over the desk, and told her how horrible I felt about the last visit and how I thought Doctor's actions were pretty fucked. She looked at me and came around the counter to give me a hug, and told me that she understood and bore no malice.

I would assume that in those days, and with Doctor having a big gay clientele, she frequently saw the after-effects of men coming out of that doctor's office. Many who would be extremely emotional.

The tears started when I left the surgery. I got on my bike to ride home. I controlled myself enough to get into the supermarket, thinking that I probably just looked really stoned. All I could think to buy was a big block of cashew chocolate and a packet of Tim Tams. I paid for my stash and got back on my bike.

It is about four kilometres to Suffolk Park where my little rented apartment was. I opened the door and shut it behind me I drew the curtains and howled.

* * *

A few months before, I had been introduced to Louise Hays' book, "You Can Heal Your Life", which I thought after reading it made some sense, but felt it was a bit wishy-washy in other respects. It was a book that was well-read on the HIV/gay scene. Some friends of mine affectionately called her 'Auntie Lou-Lou', and that name did seem to suit her. She was like a wise, old auntie who had been through her own journey and come out the other side.

The premise of this book, one of the first self-help best sellers, was that your thought patterns about self could manifest in your body as illnesses. How you thought about yourself affected your physical health. This could sit comfortably if you have a pimple or a cold sore, but this was a life threatening condition that I had. Did I really attract this bug into my life? Did my negative self-image and low esteem issues really come to this?

I ate most of the chocolate I bought after my diagnosis and started to re-read her book.

Over the next few days the tears just flowed. I thought of my life and how there had been a lot of crappy things that had happened. My school life I had hated. Not a day went by in primary or secondary school where I wasn't assaulted – either verbally or physically – about being a poofter. Had I really brought this vile disease into my life? Was I ultimately responsible for this? Should I go religious and thank all those priests for not giving me adequate protection in the schoolyard? Could I forgive those school bullies because they didn't know much better?

It took a long time for me to realise I am in control of my life and, yes, I am responsible for everything that happens in it – both the good and the not so good. Sometimes it's just a matter of perspective. School life definitely fell into the not so good or as I like to phrase it: '*School was a life challenge.*'

If I died tomorrow, would I be happy with what's gone down in my life? Would I be able to say that I was content to go if it happened to be tomorrow?

Definitely not! I don't want to die unfulfilled and disillusioned. I asked myself: 'What do I want or need to do, that would make me happier if my departure was tomorrow or next week?'

My younger sister Majella lived on the Gold Coast. She was coming down to tell me some news. I rang her and asked if she could come down as soon as possible. She came down the next day with her gorgeous boyfriend and the announcement that she was going to accept this man's offer of marriage. I had thought this was going to happen, and had been prepared with a bottle of Moet. It seemed like a good time to be extravagant. My diagnosis had happened on a Monday. I had been dismissed from my job on the previous Friday.

We toasted to her news. I was so happy for her. Then, she asked me what was so urgent. I told them both ... and then felt like an arsehole. I felt bad because Majella was going to tell Mum and Dad her fabulous news – and I intended at some stage to tell them mine. But I didn't want to rain on their parade ... I started to sense the irony of life's highs and lows. Never do these ironies or life lessons seem to string themselves out; they land on top of you all at once.

The next person I needed to talk to was Shane; a larger than life character, whose manner was gentle and understanding. He had also been in my situation. I first met Shane at Gretel Farm on an Edna Walling's tree planting day. The idea was to throw stones over your head and plant trees or seedlings where the stones fell to give a sense of randomness to the planting that is like that of the bush; not formal in any way. Shane's partner Michael was living at Gretel Farm which was owned by Chris. We hit it off instantly with a strong devotion to food. At the time we met he was living in Federal but at the time of my diagnosis he had already moved to Brisbane. He got the nickname "Auntie Shane" as he has a strong identity with family and he has a lot of the finest attributes that a mother should have. He always makes sure everyone is fed and we, his loved friends, know he has strong shoulders to cry on.

When I told him my news, Shane got on a bus from Brisbane and was at my place within a few hours. To be able to have the emotional support of a friend around was so important.

I had a "sort of" partner at the time: Mitchell. He was studying in Sydney and came up on holidays. I really was in love with this guy – or thought I was. The school year just happened to finish a few days after my diagnosis, which was November 28th. Mitchell arrived at my flat on December 2nd.

He was all bubbly at first, but when I told him my news he called me a slut. Then he accused Shane of giving me HIV (Shane and I had never even had sex).

Shane left, asking me if I wanted to go back to Brisbane with him. I decided against. I later regretted that decision.

Mitchell had had a few drinks before he arrived. Alcohol and not-so-good news are never a good combination. A tirade of abuse just seemed not to end. 'I've been so good, and here you are slutting around picking up anything!' He told me.

It went on and on. For some reason, I put this performance down to shock and forgave him. He was quite a tall man and as Eartha Kitt says on her live album: 'Where ever he went, I hope he shrank.' I do love that line!

Even though he wasn't the best person (in hindsight) to have around me at the time, he was someone – and at this stage, I seemed to be living in a state of shock. My focus became me, and coming to terms with the news. Mitchell became a schoolyard bully that I disconnected from. Although abusive, his violent streak hadn't surfaced yet, so I thought his apology was genuine. I had a lot more on my plate than he could grasp. What did I really want to do?

After the first couple of days had gone by, I came to the decision that I wanted to have the beach summer holiday of my youth. The one that I'd never had. Due to the circumstances, it seemed an appropriate course of action.

With no job (but I did get a payout), I was put on six months sickness benefits, so I had some money coming in. I paid three months of rent, put money towards the electricity and hit the beach.

I rode my pushbike everywhere and just concentrated on the "here and now". I made bread just about every day and concentrated on eating well.

* * *

Ivana's Bread

It needs to be a really good work out for you. If there's any stress issues in your life it's a really good time to make bread. For me it's really good therapy for the soul.

1 kg plain flour
   50gm of fresh yeast or two sachets of dried
   3 teaspoons of sugar
   1 teaspoon of salt
   1 tablespoon of oil
   3 cups of warm water

- Dissolve sugar in the water and then add yeast
- Add oil
- Mix into flour and knead well (this means that you need to stretch it and bring it back in on itself over and over again on a floured bench)
- You can do this stage and the following proving in the bowl or on a bench. You need to keep adding a few tablespoons of flour at a time until

the dough forms a tight ball. Punch it, pound it and give it a good beating! It needs to be a really good work out for you
- Cover with plastic wrap or a damp, clean tea towel
- Prove once (which means it needs to go somewhere warm and double in size)
- Once it's big and full of air, bash back to a firm tight dough. You may need to add a bit of flour to the dough again to keep it tight and not sticky
- Make rolls or loaves, and prove again
- Once it has achieved this stage coat the bread with an egg wash which is a yolk with a splash of milk (you could sprinkle seeds like poppy, sesame, cumin, fennel on top) and bake in a hot oven at about 220C
- The bread is cooked when you tap it and it has a hollow sound and feels light. It will take at least ¾ hour to bake two loaves from this recipe.

So in this recipe I have replaced the water with half water half tomato puree, I used other liquids like half water half wine, chicken stock, anything that had a flavour instead of just water. On the second prove when you have shaped the dough and are getting ready to be baked I have rolled the dough with a pesto or a tapenade to make a pinwheel effect. I have also added olives, anchovies, sun or semi dried tomatoes, chopped herbs or many different spices literally any sort of flavour. The only thing to consider when adding flavour is not making the dough too wet so it's too sticky to manage it well.

***

Muffins

    500gm SR Flour
    150gm melted butter
    2 beaten eggs
    4 dessertspoons of sugar (depending on flavour)
    Pinch of salt
    Approximately 1½ cups milk (any sort; cows, soy, almond etc)

- Add the milk, eggs and butter to flour, salt and sugar and till right consistency (the right consistency means "wetter than scone drop," an old Mama I used to work with, Jean Bourke would say. She got me my first hospitality job in 1978 washing dishes at the Motel Waverley – Candles Restaurant. "Wetter than scone drop" would be comparable to a sloppy pure cream; scoop out a spoonful, turn the spoon to its side and see what happens. It probably should stay for a bit on the spoon and possibly do a 'flop' onto the surface below. Experiment a few times! A scone dough should if dropped from a height, sort of, stay in the same shape. So if the dough is wetter when dropped, it wouldn't hold a shape)
- This recipe can be a base for your creativity. Like the bread recipe this can have berries or most fruit. You can replace some of the milk with some other liquid like wine or berry puree. The volume of fluid is the most important thing. Remember: if you substitute, you may have variations on texture as well

- Pour blobs into patty cases or muffin moulds and bake about 180C for about ½ hour or firm to the touch. If you have a really hot oven with a dodgy temperature you may need to turn it down for a while to maybe 150C – especially if it looks like it's getting too much colour too quickly.

* * *

Soda Bread

This is firm solid bread that's a good addition to a cold winters night stew. There's no proving or second bashings to this one.

750gm plain flour
1 teaspoon of bicarb soda
1 teaspoon of salt
½ pint (300ml) of buttermilk, sour milk, or fresh milk with a teaspoon of cream of tartar

- Mix dry ingredients together in a bowl
- Form a well (meaning from the centre of the bowl dig a hole with your fist into the dry ingredients)
- Pour liquid into centre of your well
- Mix slowly, incorporating all the flour
- Knead till dough is soft and smooth
- Flatten it out until about 5 or 6cm high circle (whatever shape)
- Cut a criss-cross into loaf
- Bake at 200C for 45 minutes.

***

Hot Onion Bread

This is from Mrs Rowe, who is a friend of mine's mother. I met her at Garth's 50th birthday and it is an old recipe of hers. She had written out the recipe for me on a piece of paper. Like many other recipes I've been given, I've kept the original hand written notes as keepsakes. After she had passed away several years back, I was going through things for this book and found Mrs Rowe's recipe. I gave it back to Garth which he was delighted to have.

This bread is great as a quick bread, and you can just about add anything to it from anchovies to grilled zucchini and everything in between. The only addition to this is I cook the onions first by chopping them up and putting into a pot with a lid. First get the heat high with a splash of olive oil, then when they start to sizzle turn the temperature to medium and cook for further 10 to 15 minutes. Let it cool before using in the dough.

500gm SR Flour
   ½ teaspoon salt
   150gm sliced onion
   60gm melted butter
   300ml sour cream or milk

- Sift flour and add 2/3 of the chopped onion
- Add butter and sour cream or milk to make a soft dough
- Knead the dough well
- Make into a large roll about 30cm long

- Brush with milk and lay remainder of onion on top
- Place on lightly floured scone tray (baking tray)
- Bake at 190C until golden and crusty
- Approx 30-40 minutes
- Serve hot. Its good toasted at a later date as well.

* * *

Belle's Damper

Damper is something that can be really bad, and it's rarely fabulous. It is possibly one of the few baked goods that doesn't need a recipe. All it requires is self-raising flour, water and salt as the essentials. My preferences, more than essentials, are a camp oven, an open fire and patience. One of the most amazing things I've ever tasted was a chocolate damper made at Confest in a fire pit, in a camp oven by Belle.

A gorgeous woman with a mass of curls on her head appeared with her camp oven and asked if she could cook her damper. I said the only condition is I get a piece. She smiled and said that was fine. I suppose I wasn't expecting much from the end result. I hadn't even asked her till it was just about cooked, about an hour later, what her recipe was. Belle told me it was a pumpkin, feta, roast capsicum damper. This got my curiosity going and when she lifted the lid the smell was magnificent.

The incredible feeling of having my pre conceived presumptions blown so far out of the water is a buzz. She obviously was a master at her craft. She used flour, into which she had put last night's mashed pumpkin, chopped roasted capsicums and made dough. To this she hand rolled through some feta cheese. It was sealed tight in the camp oven. Baking paper layers between dough and lid and foil was used to seal the lid.

This was then placed on the edge of the burning coals. With a shovel she dropped some coals on top of the lid. About three quarters of an hour later she returned checked it and gave it a little while longer then when it was ready she offered me some. It was exquisite!

The next day she blew my mind more with a chocolate, marinated-dried fruit damper with a toffee crust. This is on my list titled "the best things I've ever eaten."

Approximately, the ratio for a sweet damper is ¾ of a cup sweetener to 500gm of flour.

You can add sugar (white, brown or raw) to the flour and either or; honey, golden syrup, molasses, pear juice concentrate etc. to the base to get to a slightly sticky dough.

To this dough Belle added chopped chocolate and dried fruit that had marinated in orange juice. When the dough was at the right consistency, she put brown sugar on top and sealed the oven. The sugar had gone to a glorious toffee. The "bread" itself was beautiful and of a lovely stretchy texture.

When baking in my camp oven, I use a cake tin, which fits snugly in the oven. Between the tin and the base of the oven I place two of three stones of a similar height to diffuse the direct heat from oven to tin.

I have also had a good damper where yoghurt was used as the liquid. Again it was really lovely. I can remember eating fabulous damper at Confest but I sometimes feel guilty that I can't remember the names of half of my friends that have passed away.

* * *

START WITH YOUR OWN ONION

Banana Bread
250gm banana
250gm sugar
2 eggs
110ml milk
55ml oil
250gm flour
5gm salt
10gm bicarb of soda

- Combine all ingredients by pureeing bananas and adding everything to a cake batter consistency
- Pour batter into a cake or loaf tin that has been lined with baking paper
- Bake in a moderate oven till firm to touch; approximately 1 hour.

This lasts for ages in the fridge and freezes well. Great served with soft cheese or as a cake with buttery icing in its own right. You can add dried fruit and nuts to the batter as well.

* * *

December 1993

All the things that I had done and those that I wanted to do – ideas and some forgotten memories – came bubbling up, and would just jump into my brain.

I was sitting on the beach just watching the waves come in and it occurred to me that I had not seen most of the Disney cartoon movies. They definitely went on the list. So this became the start of an almost non ending bucket list. A list of things like this should be as long as it needs to be. There would be no restrictions on the number of items. Certainly there was travel, money and success that were on the imagined list, but things that took a priority were the ones that were within my reach.

Suffolk Park in those days was pretty much full of alternative-lifestyle people and locals that had done very well with the increase in land values. The small community had a pub, a fish and chip shop, a video shop and a general store – all across the road from my unit. That night after being at the beach for most of the day, I went over to the video store and got out Fantasia and Beauty and the Beast. For the next week or so, I watched all that the video shop had.

I thought of all the things that I hadn't done: skydiving, scuba diving – and because I was a chef: the foods I hadn't eaten. Adventure sports scared the crap out of me. As for food, I settled my mind on the thought that I'd done most of it.

My apprenticeship at The Queenscliff Hotel almost ten years before had given me every gourmet luxury that one could imagine to the point that I believe I overdosed on luxury. I'd made and tasted Krug champagne sorbet, beluga caviar on blinis, seafood of all shapes and sizes. What was normally spent by a customer on one meal for one person was the entire budget for feeding three hundred people at a soup kitchen in St Kilda I had done some volunteering at.

While I was working at Queenscliff we heard that the famous Two Faces was closing (which was a big deal). The owners were taking over an old convent on the Mornington Peninsula. Poaching of some staff from Queenscliff started happening soon after the closure of Two Faces.

Patricia, the owner of Queenscliff, Ross and I were

talking about the closure. She offered to pay for Ross; another chef John, and myself to go on the last night. Well, we thought that we were going to have a good night by ourselves but we arrived to find that there were three other guests.

Virginia Hellier (a hospitality industry consultant), Rita Erlich (a food critic for The Age, Good Food Guide) and Mietta (Patricia's sister) who was a famous restaurateur in her own right. I remember three things: one; a nashi pear conversation, they were a new fruit and I recall them costing about four or five dollars each.

Two; the dessert I chose was chestnut spaghetti, which wasn't very nice.

And three; Patricia rang during the meal and each of us men went to the phone to say our thanks. I was last and had had a few drinks. I said to her: 'You have led three lambs to the slaughter.' That's how formidable these women were.

* * *

The best meal I have ever had was a crayfish mousseline wrapped in brioche with a Pernod and bisque sauce made by the best chef I have ever had the pleasure to work with.

Michael was muscled, handsome and I was a bit infatuated with him. He was married with a beautiful wife and children, so I knew my infatuation was just that (and that he was undeniably heterosexual was the other major complication!). Most of Michael's charm was that he was so talented and knowledgeable about food. Every day was a learning experience.

1988 Queenscliff Victoria

I remember the days when the fishermen would come into the kitchen. Some, in the earlier years, were men who had just caught too much and tried to offload their catches by selling to the chefs at the local hotels. As the Fisheries department got stronger in regulations these guys became less frequent.

Gus, a licensed fisherman, was a big weathered man with a huge handlebar moustache. He caught crays when in season as well as snapper and yellowtail for a living.

The crays were brought into the kitchen in large hessian potato sacks. The tuna, almost four to five feet high, would be put on hooks and hung in the cool room. To the untrained person this was a bit of a gruesome sight to see; sometimes six huge fish that had been gutted and hung in the cool room. One Christmas time Tony, a quite effeminate man and one of the very professional group of waiters in the dining room, walked in and all we heard was a drop of trays and a huge scream. We ran in to find Tony hunched over the sink in the scullery, cursing the chefs as no one had prepared him for the macabre sight.

We learnt that we had to cut a little piece from the yellowtails tail and cook it as sometimes the flesh was all mushy. I'm not sure why that happened, but it was a bitch if you didn't do it and prepared the huge fish for service and only during service would you find out that it was not good.

This was the first time I had made brioche and a cooked mousseline. I had Michael's undivided attention for a while, so together we made the crayfish mousseline wrapped in brioche. I killed the crays with a knife length ways through the centre of the animal then washed the brainy bits and took out the flesh (still pulsing a bit).

Because there are two different processes to this meal it was also a lesson in time management by combining the tasks or stages of the different processes. Brioche dough has stages similar to bread making and needs time so it's of use. The mousse needs to be prepared and par-cooked before it's wrapped in the brioche and baked.

By about four o'clock in the afternoon we pulled out this beautiful creation from the oven. The shells of the crayfish were used to make the Pernod and bisque sauce. I really was in heaven. I had "God" all to myself for most of the day – and here we were sampling this magnificent creation. We were standing in the servery area of the kitchen eating a slice, with a glass of wine that we had got from Ross, the headwaiter (in exchange for a slice for himself), talking about textures and combining flavours feeling really proud of this dish. Michael was praising the end result and then the scream from the scullery happened.

The kitchen was a large room with a long servery. The scullery was a separate room at the opposite end of the kitchen further on was the cool room. Even before having a chance to react to the scream, Eileen Butler, our much loved kitchen hand, came running into the kitchen and straight into my arms. She was hysterical. For a few seconds, we didn't know what to do. I just held her in my arms as her screams and sobs continued.

'My son is dead. No, no, no, no,' were the words that came out of her mouth.

'Who has gone Eilly? Oh, darling.' With that, Eileen's daughter, Trish, walked in with tears in her eyes. She told us what she had just relayed to her mother.

He was in Tasmania. A fisherman – and, it being his birthday, had been celebrating. It was the last time he had been seen. No one knew how, but the police found his body in the sea a few days later. His death was determined as accidental.

Eileen, at that time, had worked at the hotel for over twenty years. She knew the hotel inside out and was loved and respected by everyone. Every chef that went through the hotel knew if Eileen was on your shift you never had to worry. Floors were clean, vegetables prepared and surfaces shone. She smoked Escorts and was always good to borrow a smoke from.

The talks that we had together out on the back steps with a ciggie and coffee are some of my most treasured moments at the hotel. Generally I would have some piece of cake or ice cream, biscuit or chocolate that I had made and she was my tester. So with coffee, fag and sweet, we would solve the world's problems or gossip about the latest crazy thing that had happened. I never saw her as an older woman. I saw her as a friend; a very special friend.

She commented one day that before she died she would like to go to the opera. We went to see The Pearl Fishers then walked up Bourke Street after the show and saw the Myer Christmas windows. We had pre and post show drinks at Mietta's and she told me it was one of the best nights of her life. She hadn't been to Melbourne for about 20 years before then.

Eileen was the first woman, first friend; I was honoured and privileged to be part of a mother's grief over the loss of her son. I couldn't speak much, for the tears had started to flow from me. I will never, to this day, forget the screams that came from Eileen. The tragedy sent lofty talk of food and slightly gushing admiration out the window and levelled us all.

An hour or so later, when we had sort of got it together, Eilly went home. We had to work on. The world stops for no one. It is one of the hardest things to do sometimes to just keep on going when all you want to do is curl up into a ball because life is too hard.

* * *

How many sons since then have I seen go to God? Sometimes I feel it's like a saying or proverb because of how easily it seems to roll off my tongue: 'I stopped counting at over eighty funerals.'

Most people just look at me incredulously. I recall the first time I met a gay man who was of a similar age to me who said he had not seen or known anybody to die of AIDS. I looked him in the eyes and said: 'How long have you been out of the closet? Twenty seconds?'

He did try to convince me that it had been longer. Amazingly, there are many people who never saw any of the horror. It was at this time that I came to the conclusion that the term "Gay Community" didn't mean anything about a united group of people with similar beliefs and ideals. It is all just genetic stuff. That's the only link. Was it GaGa that said: 'Born this way'?

My belief is that the people who died of the virus are heroes and martyrs; especially those that took medications or had treatments, whether scientific or alternative, that were experimental. In the early days of medication I was prescribed nearly 40 pills a day. This caused more diarrhoea and vomiting than I could conceive was humanly possible. When so much stuff comes out of your body and not much goes in it's hard to imagine where it comes from. I had it very easy compared to others though. Because I lived.

It is this sort of history, in my observation, that a lot of young people in the GLBTIQ community have no idea of. Without these people trying out experimental ideas and drugs the positive people on medication today would not be here. Science has learnt from the numbers game.

It is a perception that gays are supposed to be sympathetic. Unfortunately I find it hard to get past some of the "community's" superficiality. When I first came out the gay newspapers seemed to be full of politics and HIV/AIDS material. Now, on the odd occasion I look, gay magazines seem to be full of the latest beauty techniques, the body beautiful, waxing, Botox, makeup, real estate and little else. The only politics is around marriage and, unfortunately, that has overtaken any other issues – like suicide numbers in young men, mental and physical health and drug and alcohol issues.

There are quite a few people who have lived with the virus for twenty years or more. Some positive people have been fortunate enough to have had few side effects or a not-so-strong virus – or a better immune response. They have been able to carry on and work and still play the game. But there are lots that are living with a post-traumatic stress.

This war was not fought overseas in some faraway land that we could conveniently watch on the news; it was a war in which young men died horribly right in front of us. A lot of these mainly men were treated appallingly by society, their families, health professionals, and anyone who became included in the knowledge that "He had AIDS."

One of the main reasons I left Melbourne in 1992 was because my whole collection of male friends, excluding two, had died. Standing at the bar of the Exchange Hotel one night, I surveyed the people and I realised I didn't know a face. Six months before I would have known at least ten faces on any particular night. It was time to get out of Melbourne. If I was going to be a stranger anywhere it had to be in a different place where I was a stranger. Not here in my home town.

* * *

Brioche

    50gm yeast
    4 ½ cups of flour
    ½ cup sugar
    8 tablespoon room-temperature soft butter
    10 yolks and 2 whole eggs
    1 cup milk

- This is made similar to bread: flour sugar together, make a well
- Add yeast to the milk then gradually add to the well
- Eggs are added to the dough
- Then the room temperature butter
- Both the dough and butter need to be of a similar temperature because if the dough is warmer the butter wont incorporate properly
- Dough needs to prove like bread: twice
- The second prove, shape and let rise
- This recipe can be sweetened or used as a savoury item.

* * *

Crayfish Mousseline

    300gm crayfish
    150ml cream
    Salt, pepper and nutmeg

Fennel, dill or spring onions

- Puree cray and add cream and seasoning till just mixed
- Take out of processor and fold through chopped fennel, dill or spring onions
- The mixture is then wrapped in glad wrap to form a tight sealed tube
- Then placed into simmering water and the tube is poached, turning when needed. This is done till slightly firm to touch
- Once that is cooked it is taken out of the liquid and left for a few minutes to cool
- In a tin lined with brioche (matching size for cray mousse) the mousse is placed in the tin wrapped with brioche
- Let the brioche prove and bake till golden brown.

***

Bisque Sauce

This sauce can be made into a soup by adding more stock and if you run out of that then some white wine or champagne can be used to thin it out. The shells used can be any crustacean – the same method is used. When it's Christmas and there are lots of prawns around, I like to utilise the prawn heads and shells to make a stock that can be frozen.

- Shells of the crayfish are smashed in the pot sautéed with onions, bay leaves and garlic

- When the water (or fish stock) is added: cook for about an hour or so, then strain
- Next a roux is made. So about 50gm butter melted in a pot, add flour till it gets "sandy" (butter and flour). Cook it for a few minutes, but be careful not to brown it too much
- Add stock slowly and stir rapidly, tomato paste can also be added at this stage
- Strain the stock and cook, adding a good splash of Pernod at the end.

* * *

Plain Batter

225gm flour (SR flour will give a little lift to the end result)

110gm butter

14gm sugar

Pinch salt

200ml water (can use beer, Guinness or cider depending on what you're doing)

- Combine together and let sit for at least half an hour
- To this you can add little, none or a whole heap of different things like mustards, chopped olives, or a bit of olive paste, sun dried tomatoes, pine nuts, chopped herbs, spring onions or garlic – anything to give the end result a bit more flavour
- Coat whatever you are using in a light dust of flour and dip into batter then into hot oil fry till golden.

* * *

Choux Pastry
 1 cup water
 50gm butter
 1 cup flour

- Combine butter and water into a pot and melt, bring to the boil and add flour, stirring constantly
- Cook till mixture comes away from the sides of pot
- When cool, add 3-4 eggs
- Pipe onto tray in desired shape and before baking splash with a little water
- Bake in a hot oven 200C till puffed and brown.

* * *

Tempura Batter
 ½ cup cornflour
 ½ cup SR flour
 ½ cup beer
 ½ cup ice water and some ice cubes

- Combine ingredients
- Let stand for a 15 minutes

* * *

When I had my first restaurant I entered the local show with five cakes. I was slightly disheartened to discover when the judging had been done that my chocolate cake was

START WITH YOUR OWN ONION

disqualified. I asked the judge why this had happened. She said: 'Well it's not a cake – it's a mousse, silly!

'Madam, it's 40 degrees in this shed; how the bloody hell would a mousse still be standing?'

She looked at me rather perplexed and said: 'So it is a cake?'

'Yes madam. It is a cake.'

I decided that the old girls didn't really like "ring-ins" – as I obviously was, because my orange cake didn't get a mention either. That cake *'had a funny texture.'*

'Madam, Claudia Roden's flourless orange cake is a middle eastern favourite.'

I didn't bother entering again when I saw that the winners had been the same winners for 40 years and the only changes happened when one of the old girls went to God and their daughters took up the challenge.

I'm not bagging these people, but maybe they were a bit inflexible in their judging. Perhaps a flourless chocolate cake that was like a mousse and a flourless almond and orange cake were just a bit too left of centre for the time.

Anyway, I have sold many serves of these cakes and the chocolate cake was Max's favourite – possibly my favourite as well. It fits all criteria: chocolate, boozy and rich! I had the pleasure to cook it for him a few times.

If you don't have a good oven and you want to make it, may I suggest getting on the phone and tracking down a friend who has a fan forced one. Make sure you bring over a bottle of wine or a few beers whilst it cooks and cools.

I've used home brand chocolate for this recipe when I have been poor and orange juice instead of the alcohol. Even if not done in a fan forced oven, it still can come out pretty damn good.

* * *

Flourless Chocolate Cake
½ lb butter
225gm chocolate
2 tablespoons milk
¼ lb almond meal
6 tablespoons castor sugar
6 eggs, separated

BEFORE STARTING THE MIXING: line the cake tin with baking paper and prepare a bain-marie (a large roasting tray that the cake tin will fit in with hot water in it. Make sure not to overfill with water). Have the bain-marie hot and in the oven when you put the cake into the tray.

- Melt the chocolate, butter and milk together
- Separately whisk the yolks and 5 tablespoons of sugar together till light in colour and well combined
- Add the chocolate mix to the beaten yolks and sugar
- Fold the almond meal through
- In another separate bowl, whisk the whites till light and fluffy adding the last tablespoon of sugar and keep whipping till sugar is dissolved
- Fold ¼ of the whipped whites through the chocolate mix till well combined then fold through the rest
- Pour mix into the cake tin and bake in a moderate oven in a bain-marie for 35 to 45 minutes

- Cake is baked when it feels firm when lightly touched in the centre
- Let it stand till cool before upending onto a plate.

* * *

Similar (but with a touch of flour) Chocolate Cake

200gm chocolate
200gm butter
120gm plain flour
½ cup cocoa
1 cup of juice or brandy or your favourite liqueur
6 eggs
120gm caster sugar

- Melt the chocolate and butter together
- Then add the sugar, saving a little bit for the egg whites
- Followed by the flour, cocoa, booze or juice and egg yolks
- Combine until it is all smooth
- Whisk the whites in a separate bowl till stiff gradually adding the remaining sugar
- Fold in ½ the whites then fold through the rest. It is important to make sure this mixture is warm when you are adding the whites
- Once they are combined into a lined cake tin, cook in a bain-marie in a medium oven for about ¾ of an hour until it is firm to the touch
- Don't use a spring form tin. You have to use a solid one-piece tin. If you use something not so

high and wide cook no longer than ¾ of an hour. If your tin is deep and not so wide you may need to cook for one to one and a half-hours.

* * *

Max said it was the cake that made him better – and for a time he certainly was.

I made the cake for him quite a few times. He liked to pull it out of the fridge when guests arrived and say that he had just whipped it up. I let him have that.

For the last six months of Max's life he needed full time care. Martin and I assisted in the duties that needed to be done. At one stage, Max had to go into hospital and he wanted me to move into his house to look after it while he was away. The lease had expired on my flat so I gave notice and moved into Max's place.

During his time in hospital, Mitchell had come back for the holidays. Max was fine with both of us there until a few days after he had returned home. Mitchell decided to get drunk and violent. Max was in his television room out of harm's way. As I was thrown against furniture and paintings on the wall, Mitchell punched and screamed at me.

I needed to get him out of the house for Max's sake, so I ran outside and he followed. Out on the street he became the Wicked Witch in Sleeping Beauty; larger than life. The situation was incomprehensible. A tirade of abuse was being hurled at me in a dying man's home.

'What the fuck are you doing here looking after this AIDS-ridden faggot? Especially when you are going to go that way too?' It went on and on. I managed to get inside and lock him out.

Through the door I said: 'If you don't fuck off I'm calling the police.' With that, another wave of verbal abuse came at the house.

'You sick fucks are going to die. Greg Kelly takes it up the arse and he's got AIDS.'

'I mean it Mitchell. I'm calling the cops.'

With that, he got into his car and drove off at high speed. I really hoped he would wrap himself around a pole or at least get done by the police. After he had sped off, I turned to look at Max's house and wanted to vomit. The door to the television room opened tentatively. Max's face appeared and he asked if I was okay. I looked at him and with tears in my eyes said: 'Yes. Unfortunately, that can't be said of your home.'

We were both in a state of shock. He asked me what had happened and, to this day, I still don't know.

All that I could do during this onslaught of savagery was just try and protect myself. The fact I was in a dying man's home was paramount in my head. I couldn't respond with force. It was impossible for me to get violent or retaliate so close to a dying man.

I started to clean up. I took the framed things that had broken off the wall and put them in the garage. I collected broken cups and got the vacuum and went over the floor. There hadn't been too much damage done to the walls that a little bit of filler wasn't going to fix. By the time I had finished and sat down Max looked at me and said: 'Fuck, love! How hard did he hit you? The bastard!'

The look on Max's face unsettled me enough to go and look in the bathroom mirror. What I saw was not the best I've ever looked. As I followed the shape of my nose, which now went a different direction to when I last looked at it that morning, I also realised my right hand throbbed. On inspection, I guessed that he had broken my thumb and, by the looks of it, my nose.

In the bedroom where we had been sleeping I saw all my record and CD collection scattered over the floor. They looked like they had been jumped on. They *had* been jumped on. *Bastard!* I thought.

Max came in and looked over my shoulder. 'Love, I don't want to tell you what to do with your life, but he can't live here.'

I replied: 'I am so humiliated. I can't believe anyone could do this to anyone else let alone someone else's home. Let alone your house. Have no fear, he isn't going to be here anymore.' With that, I grabbed all of Mitchell's belongings and put them out next to the garbage bin on the street.

I felt as if I had created this horrible mess in Max's life and I needed to give him some space as well.

The next day Mitchell came by with the biggest grovelling act. Flowers and apologies, telling me that he didn't want to break up and *blahh, blahh, blahh!* He spoke of the stress he was under at university and he did not know what had overcome him. At this stage, I might add, he was studying physiotherapy.

Suffice to say, I forgave him and we found an apartment that afternoon in Byron.

Within two weeks, he had another go with a similar situation - one minute fine, the next off his rocker. We were getting out of the car when it started. I was under the garage door and I'd bent down to get something and suddenly the garage roll-a-door, with no padding on its end, came down furiously on my back. My first thought was that my back had been broken, but I found I could move. I ran up the stairs to get into the flat, but he pushed his way in. It started.

But this time was different. This time I was in my territory and I punched back.

He had grabbed a mop and started to whack me with it. I snatched it out of his hands as it hit my chest. I have never really been violent, but this night it wasn't just Mitchell I was hitting. I hit every motherfucker that had given me grief in my life. With a surprising amount of force that overcame me, I turned from being a victim to someone who stood up for themselves – and boy did it feel good!

His pleas to stop hurting him still, I have to admit, made me smile. It sounds terrible, but it is the truth. With about two whacks from the mop handle after I had got it out of his hands, my thumb broken again, and about four punches from me it was over.

'You've broken my rib you bastard!'

'Mitchell, I'm leaving now. You can have this place; your name is on the lease. I'm gone.'

'You can't leave me with this. I don't have any money!'

'You think I care, arsehole?'

'I'll leave ... and find somewhere else tomorrow,' he pleaded. With that I started to pack my clothes 'What are you doing?'

'I said I'm out of here now, or you are out of here now. I am not having you in my face for another night.'

After pleas, grovels, apologies and *'it won't happen again'* he was gone.

I went over to his wall cabinet and thought of all my CD's that he'd jumped on. CD's were a real comfort; an indulgence during the sadness and grief throughout this time. There were too many to replace; possibly 80 of my favourites. The others that weren't so bad had been put in storage. It was just a savage thing to do but, for whatever reason, he did do it. He obviously didn't think very highly of me.

I opened the door of Mitchell's collection of boxed crystal glasses an assortment of presents he'd received over his life. Gifts that were given by Auntie-whomever or any other person who blew their money giving this guy a gift and I grabbed the first box. The stingy side of me said: *'Don't be wasteful ...'* the vengeful side of me said: *'Party!'* Vengeful won that very quick debate.

I placed open palms on either side of the box and held it firmly. I was aware of this hatred growing in me. I did not want to hang on to it. This is the state of mind that gets you sick. This emotion becomes a presence in your life and feeds on negativity. I knew that this anger needed to be exorcised because if it didn't it would kill me. I'd been positive for about a year it was still early days there was no treatment. To have a burning passionate hate for him was only going to take my energy and serve it to him on a plate. *He is not going to ruin my life!*

I was in pain; I'd been humiliated, physically and emotionally abused, and manipulated. It was a reverential bang on the floor each box received. The glass smashing inside could almost have been a musical instrument. It was a great sound! I heard that lovely sound about a dozen times that day. As I repeated the process, I felt my spirits lift higher with each box I grabbed.

Once, forgiveness was the appropriate thing to do. Twice – for my own self-worth – I forgave myself for putting myself in that situation, accompanied by learning the lesson.

There is a standard of behaviour that I expect from people, especially those that I get intimate with. Mitchell showed me clearly what I will accept and what I won't. The distance between what I will and will not accept used to be a grey area, but thanks to him there is a clear line in the sand in my life.

I went to Max's house the next day he looked at me and told me to get in the car as we were going to the doctor. About a month later (nose back in place, black eyes and bruises diminished, broken thumb healing) I rode my push-bike to Suffolk Park to see Max. This ride had become a daily ritual. Max's health was going down fast. Martin met me at the front door and gave me some sandwiches that he had prepared and said that I was to have a day off; that Max was having a good day and I should go to the beach.

I went in to say hello to Max and he said in a soft, campy voice dripping in sarcasm: 'Love, fuck off. Leave me alone. See if I care.'

I knew he was having a go, and I just laughed. He smiled too and I gave him a kiss, said my farewells and went to Braes Beach, my most favourite place on the planet.

* * *

Mick Hannan loved a roast. He did it well too. When you were invited for dinner the cooked meal was put on the bench. On a chopping board sat a piece of meat or whole chook with roasted vegies in the tray and gravy made in a jug. You were to cut off as much meat as you wanted, plate up yourself and sit on the couch where Mick generally held court.

He had an old wood oven that was only used as a heater and his old gas stove would produce the dinner. When the meal was finished his ritual of giving Tommy (Mick's Labrador) the plates to lick clean didn't thrill me. I don't have a love connection with an animal like that. I have other friends that do but when I finish I generally go straight to the sink to rinse my plate. I don't know where it comes from. In the early years of HIV there was some issue with parvo virus being contagious from kittens and pups. Dogs and cats have their place, but not at the table. If I tried to get on my knees and have a go at getting something from the dogs bowl I'm sure the dog would bite me. So I play by the dog rules!

I met Mick in the early years of my time in the Northern Rivers at one of the famous ACON retreats. I think the first, actually. These have become an institution over the last 20 years or so and I have another connection with them in the more recent years with Shane.

Mick was, I considered, to be one of the "A-gays" of the area. He lived in an old farm house that had seen better days and Mick was not one to pick up a feather duster or a vacuum cleaner, let alone use them. The old house was on a hill with a long drive way which started with a sharp turn off the road at the front gate. It was called Hazeldene and the sign at the gate was the marker of the driveway that came up rather quickly, heading to Bangalow from Clunes.

He was a very handsome man with an exuberant personality. He could be loud and get carried away within a discussion. It could seem to the uninitiated that he was bordering on being abusive but it never really was. I think what he wanted was for the person to talk with him in the same way; to be just as outraged or outrageous as he was. I often started to laugh as he got carried away on the "what if's" in a conversation and that seemed to increase the volume of his voice.

When I was living at Gretel Farm in Eureka, which wasn't very far from Mick's, he would pop in and visit. In those days my only communication was a phone up at the main house. I lived in a converted cow bails which was a rather cute but basic style of living. No toilet, phone or water when I first moved in. I was lucky to have electricity. The properties around Gretel Farm were all macadamia plantations and at harvest time the sound of the factories processing nuts was something that you got used to, but was a loud constant noise that came from about half a kilometre away.

If I got more than one or two phone calls it became bothersome for the owners to call out to me to come and answer the phone. A lot of the time people would just drop in. Many times friends would travel between Byron and Lismore and drop in on the way, to see if I wanted to go in the direction they were going.

The Bails, as it was called, was basically two rooms which consisted of a large room and the bedroom which had a lovely bay window. Both sides of the bails were glass windows and doors. The view was of the Moreton Bay fig tree on one side and the farm on the other. It sat under the huge tree which was said to be several hundred years old. It was constantly alive, or felt like it was. At different times of the year it would drop fruit on the corrugated tin roof or small branches or every once in a while the carpet snakes that lived in the tree would miss there "footing" and fall, creating a huge thud and frightening the be-Jesus out of everyone. Possums would scurry across the roof along with smaller sounding scurries which would be the rats. One of the most respected cats I've ever known was Fritz. He ate nine rats in one evening and in the morning deposited nine noses, tails and some sort of organ on the mat at the door. He waited for me, and when I awoke he meowed loudly till I acknowledged his effort. Then he went into the garden and sunshine and didn't move for hours – I think because he was so full.

Every once in a while a more interesting creature would pop its head in. Larry and Curly, two browns that I had been aware of, once came out after I had spent a long day in the garden creating beds and laying down straw and did this amazing "dance of love", interlocking their bodies in a spellbinding trance. If you've ever seen browns mating, it truly is a special thing.

I got myself inside very quickly as they did their dance and I realised I needed to call one or the other a more feminine name, but I didn't know who was who so they stayed as Larry and Curly.

Another time near to sunset, I was reading by the Ned Kelly fire box which heated the room and a huge slam banged on the glass sliding door. I looked up to see a magnificent large owl that had not seen the glass and full body-slammed the window. I leapt up and went out to see if it was okay. It was a large animal and had severe looking claws and beak. Not something I wanted to scare. I sat with it for a while; it didn't seem to have broken wings or anything just maybe in shock. I had some mince in the fridge which I left it and an egg which I cracked into a bowl. It was a beautiful bird and was unsure what to do. The only thing was to leave it till morning and see if it recovered. I was several kilometres from a phone the main house was locked up, so I made it comfortable and went to bed.

In the morning an exquisite impression of the owl in minute detail had been left on the glass. I had kept my eye on the owl and made sure the cats couldn't get to it and by morning he or she had gone.

The Bails were a romantic place to live. I had a few great parties there. One was a tree trimming party that even had a choir singing Christmas carols. There is a video of that performance somewhere – possibly not a video player to play it, though. It was the year of horrendous fires around the Northern Rivers and my idea with this style of party was for invited guests to bring a decoration, preferably handmade, and non-perishable food items. My tree gets decorated and has a beautiful bounty underneath. That year we had about four station wagons full of everything from tampons to flour, kids' Christmas pressies, to canned soup and condoms. The look on some of the volunteers' faces was priceless when they started unpacking things. Some of my friends who worked at ACON had supplied condom and lube sachets. The women didn't know where to look. Anyway, we dropped off all the goodies and felt good about it.

It was several years later that the opportunity came to pass that Mick invited me to stay in his home. I had been speaking about not having anywhere to live and he said: 'Come live with me.'

I jumped at the opportunity and moved in within days. My things went into storage and I became a bit of a free spirit. We had a chat about rent and he refused to take any money so I said that I would help cook and do the cleaning, which he agreed on. When Mick was out of the house I could move furniture and vacuum, sweep and dust. I cleared cobwebs that had been there for years. I went through the mould specimens in the pantry, checking before I threw anything out. I cleaned shelves and got the house to a standard that I was happy with. The garden was a jungle and I eventually got into it and did a major transformation over the year or so I was there.

People would come and be stunned at the state of the house. Mick would laugh and say the pixies had been. There was a time when a very handsome friend of Mick's had come to visit and they arrived back a bit early. I was on the floor scrubbing the skirting boards of the lounge room. He looked at me and said: 'What's your story? Are you like the Houseboy or something?'

I laughed and said: 'Yeah, I'm the Houseboy.'

It was at the time of the first Gulf War. Mick and I were watching TV. A Brigadier was on, conveying the latest news to Australia about the war effort. His name just happened to be Mick's full name. So I turned and looked at Mick and said: 'Well, not only am I the Houseboy, but I'm the Brigadiers Houseboy.' That became an instant brand name for me!

Long before I had moved into the house there were stories that were told by friends who would stay overnight and wake up to find cows in the house shitting and mooing. The floors had never been scrubbed. They were wooden floors and had a layer of built in dirt on them. Mick had gone to Sydney for a week or so and I was left to mind the house.

I cleared everything out of the lounge room and started scrubbing. It was a beautiful Northern Rivers sort of day and I knew I was going to destroy any clothing that I would wear, so I stripped off and scrubbed the floor with soap and a scrubbing brush and plenty of warm water. It took hours; nearly a whole day's effort, and by the end of the job I had a rich red dirt stain on my hands, knees and feet.

The sun shone in the late afternoon drying up the remnants of water and soap to illuminate wood that hadn't seen the light of day in years. Once the job was done I had a great sense of satisfaction but during the laborious process I questioned myself on why I would even start such a thing. I did the whole house over the next few days and when Mick got home I was happy that he instantly recognised that it had been done. It was funny when visitors would come over look incredulous and say: *'What the fuck happened?'*

During my time at Mick's I got a hideous side effect from my medication, a wasting disease, as well as PCP (a long winded name for a type of pneumonia). The fat and muscle just left my body. Breathing became an issue later. I have a photo of Mick, Tommy the Labrador and myself. It was taken at Mick's place and it's on my fridge as a reminder to myself of where I've been; that I have come from there to this moment in time. In the photo, I weighed 49 kilos. I'm 86 kilos now, and much healthier at 50 years old than I ever could have hoped for at 30.

When people talk about getting older and they make a negative or ageist comment, I respond that I don't believe in old age at all. I was old at 30 and I get younger every day.

* * *

Roast Beef

There are quite a few different cuts of beef that you can roast. If you're uncertain and you want something nice ask your butcher. Select what you want to roast. If it's a boneless piece I like to buy a couple of bones maybe rib bones to throw into the tray to cook the meat on. You can also roughly chop some onions, carrots and celery. Toss them in olive oil, into the tray and put the meat on that. This is to keep it off the tray and stop it from directly burning.

- First I rub olive oil onto the meat (Nana Young would have used dripping that would have been collected from previous roasts)
- A seasoned piece of meat generally means to

sprinkle liberally salt and pepper on it, do this after you've oiled
- I like to grab decent fresh sprigs of rosemary and put these with the bottom vegetables or bones to add aroma and flavour. Thyme and sage are other favourites for roasting which can be loosely chopped or broken apart and placed on top of the meat
- I don't mind stabbing small holes in the meat and inserting some herb, anchovies or whole cloves of garlic
- Put the meat into a hot oven (220C) for at least 20 minutes then turn it down to about 180C
- Allow approximately 15 minutes per 500gms of meat plus an extra 15 minutes cooking time.
- You can baste the meat a few times which means just get a big spoon and scoop up the oily juicy stuff in the tray and pour it over the meat
- I like meat to be under rather than over and to test this give it a poke with a fork if the juice comes out with a bit of blood tinge to it then you are done enough for me
- Once the time is up it needs to sit for a good twenty minutes covered and let rest before carving. This gives you enough time to make the gravy
- Place the meat on a carving tray or somewhere covered
- Put the roasted bones and or vegies into a pot set aside
- If you can easily scoop most of the fat from the tray then do so with a spoon or I like to layer a sheet at a time of paper towel over the tray to

absorb the fat lifting quickly each sheet and discarding
- The idea is to try and keep the maximum amount of the pan juices with as little of the fat. Nana Young would probably call me wasteful for discarding this precious fat or dripping.

* * *

Gravy Jus

- There's a few ways to make gravy. Grant used to put the meat on a small tray and from the baking tray discard as much of the liquid fat as possible.
- Add a good splash of Worcestershire sauce, about a glass of red wine and some water over heat bring to the boil and scrap all the caramelised bits off the tray
- When boiling, thicken with a tablespoon of corn flour dissolved in a half cup of water
- Boil the tray up making sure all the yummy goodness has left the pan's base
- If it looks too thick add some liquid to thin it down or more cornflour if too thin
- Taste the gravy and add salt and pepper.

A more traditional version (for four people):

- Leave about a tablespoon of fat in the roasting tray

- To this add 2 tablespoons of flour
- Cook this like the previous on the stove top and the fat and flour will mix together. This will stick quite quickly but make sure all the fat is mixed with the flour
- Once that is done add some stock, water or wine or all three
- Stir really well and slowly add enough liquid to remove all the caramelised bits from the pan. This needs to be cooked well so you can't taste the flour.

At this stage with both types of gravy or even if you have used the packet stuff in the tray you can add a good tablespoon of mustard (any type), chopped herbs or spring onions, caramelised onions, anchovies, pesto, tapenade, literally anything that you think will go well with the meal you are serving. The best part other than the taste of making gravy like this is that you actually make washing up much easier, by boiling all the yummy bits off there is less effort in washing up.

Essentially other meats be they veal lamb or game generally you would follow the same principle. The important thing is that meat needs to be sealed on a high heat first up. This can be done directly on a stove top, on a BBQ outside or in a hot oven. If you have a smaller piece of meat and good ventilation in your kitchen it is a relatively easy process. I have lived in a smaller flat for a long time with bad ventilation, so sealing meat on a stove top can be a little boring. On more than one occasion I have set off the fire alarm.

When making stews, casseroles cassolets or whatever

fancy name some French chef gives them, sealing your meat is the same principle.

Cubed meat, or chunks of like an osso bucco, ox tail, or even chicken chunks can be put into a freezer bag. Add a couple of tablespoons of flour to the bag with salt and pepper and any other spice or herb you like. When sealing smaller batches of the meat brown in a pot then take out and put aside.

Then add vegetables. Always add onions first and cook them well before adding carrots, celery, capsicum or any other root vegetable.

As far as I'm concerned garlic is a must which can be added as the onions are near to finished cooking. For thick hearty casseroles during winter I love whole cloves of garlic thrown in with the onions.

Once all the vegies and meat are browned then liquid is added to the pot, to boil off all the lovely caramelised residue on the bottom. This can be wine, stock, water, a pasta tomato sauce. I have even used left over pumpkin soup or other soups as a base liquid. A good splash of Guinness, beer or cider depending on the meat the options are literally endless.

When you start to pour in the liquid add a cup at a time making sure the sauce has dissolved all the flour and there are no lumps. Once this is done everything can be thrown into the pot and cooked on the stove, into a casserole dish and covered baked slowly in the oven or thrown into a crock pot and left for many hours. There is nothing nicer than doing a quick preparation in the morning and coming home to the smell of a gorgeous stew in the crock pot on a cold winter night.

* * *

GREGORY KELLY

My dear friend Shane has been a huge positive influence in my life. He has supported me through grief and trauma even whilst going through his own. I hope in some way I have been as valuable a friend to him as he always has been to me. Every time Lismore floods, my thoughts are not far away from him, his partner Neil and their dogs: Dot and Betty.

I really have done some amazing things through his generosity. I had the privilege of having a home away from home in Brisbane when I was in the Northern Rivers, I got to see some amazing concerts, and our trip to the APY Lands was a powerful and unforgettable experience.

He is an excellent chef, artist and a devoted carer when the situation has arisen. When we work together we have an excellent time. Our passion for good food is similar and when we are together we spend a lot of time laughing. One of my favourite memories is cooking with Shane at the ACON retreats. I have had the fantastic pleasure of going up to my spiritual homeland and spending a week helping to prepare menus, pick up the orders and cook for our fellow positive brothers.

Since the early days of the retreats over 20 years ago, the changes to the lives of People Living With HIV/AIDS has been dramatic. Still though, issues around isolation, disclosure, mental health and physical ailments impede many people's lives. This is why the retreats are so important.

Combined, Shane and I have been cooking for at least 60 years, so we can put on a pretty good spread. I always feel honoured to be part of the crew. A lot of energy is given to counselling whether it's organised or impromptu, therapeutic workshops or physical activities. Many conversations have happened over the kitchen sink with attendees helping out in the kitchen. Conversations are started and suddenly I'm aware that they feel comfortable enough to start talking on a deeper level. It is a responsibility that I totally respect and recognise its incredible value to many men's lives.

Not being able to talk to people in a similar situation can be detrimental to a healthy lifestyle and having a space over a long weekend where people feel safe to unburden themselves is vital.

I love at the end of the retreat when fond farewells are being shared; real friendships have been made and continue. I have met many men through this venture and ongoing friendships are a testament to the integrity of the workshops and leadership skills shown by the coordinators.

Spending time with your best friend doing what you do best: cooking, eating, laughing, sharing stories and cracking one liners at each other is, for me, one of life's joys. I am very aware that we reflect how important having good people in your life really is; how laughter and a positive outlook is essential in quality of life. When the quality and quantity of my life was at an all-time low, when I was questioning the validity of keeping on going when symptoms and side effects of medications overrode most enjoyment in life, I always knew that Shane was never far away. Shane is and has always been a truly honest, open, dear friend who has been there in my darkest hours and he is one of my angels.

This is a typical menu that Shane and I would whip up for the Northern Rivers retreats. It is said that the guys come for the food more than the content of the retreat but I do believe it's an all-round thing: the food, the people, the instructors, the place and the vibe all mix to become a fabulous experience. I always cherish cooking for it with Shane.

GREGORY KELLY

* * *

Friday, February 7, 2014

Hummus & Beetroot Dip
Antipasto, Cheese & Fresh Fruit Platters with Assorted Breads 'n' Crackers
Oven Baked Barramundi with Lemon Butter & Parsley
Arancini Balls with Mushroom, Artichoke Caper & Pesto
Steamed Minted Potatoes
Caramelised Beetroot Walnut with Goats Feta Rocket Salad

Dessert:
21st Birthday Cake Chocolate, Beetroot & Hazelnut Meal Cake
Strawberries, Cream & Ice-cream

Beverages:
Tea, Coffee, Juices, H2o

Saturday, February 8, 2014

Breakfast:
Swiss Muesli – Poached Eggs on Spinach Fruit Salad – Stewed Prunes – Yoghurt, Assorted Cereals – Milk – Soy
Toast – Brown & Mixed grain

Lunch:
Assorted Turkish Breads, Chicken – Basil Mayonnaise
Ham – Tomato – Swiss Cheese – Pickles
Egg – Lettuce
Tomato – Cheese

START WITH YOUR OWN ONION

Roasted Capsicum – Eggplant Fruit

Dinner:

Pumpkin, Sweet Potato, Spinach, Cumin Sausage Roll with Beetroot Salsa

Kangaroo, Thyme & Garlic Sausage Roll with Beetroot Salsa

Tossed Salad

Dessert:

Mixed Berry Cake with a Mixed Berry Sauce

Sunday, February 9, 2014

Breakfast:

Poached Eggs on Spinach & Bacon Assorted Cereals – Milk – Soy Fruit Salad – Stewed Prunes – Yoghurt

Toast – Brown & Mixed grain

Lunch:

Wraps – Roast Pumpkin & Hummus

Corned Silverside with Aioli

Ham & Mustard

Beetroot, Avocado & Sprouts

Fruit

Dinner:

Vegetarian Stuffed Mushrooms

Chicken Drumstick Stroganoff with North Coast Dry-Land Rice

Peach Macadamia Cake & Poached Peaches

Monday, February 10, 2014

Breakfast:
Poached Eggs on Spinach Assorted Cereals – Milk – Soy
Fruit Salad – Stewed Prunes – Yoghurt
Toast – Brown & Mixed Grain
Lunch:
BBQ – Chick Pea & Vegetable Patties
Italian & Chicken Sausages Coleslaw – Beetroot – Green
Salad Fruit
Dinner:
Stir Fry Tofu

Grilled Pork Chop & Apple Sauce

Roast Potatoes, Carrot, Peas & Beans

Panetone with Fruit Salad

Tuesday, February 11, 2014

Breakfast:
Assorted Cereals – Milk – Soy Fruit Salad – Stewed Prunes
– Yoghurt
Toast – Brown & Mixed Grain

* * *

It was Shane who rang me to tell me that Mick had died; alone, slowly, from a preventable viral (or bacterial – not sure which) meningitis. Shane has had the task of informing me of Robert's passing as well as another friend, Johnny.

Johnny was a scientist who never told anyone that he

was HIV positive as well as Hep C and did nothing about it. He lived for 20 years with these conditions which in itself is no mean feat. When he was finally hospitalised he was well and truly beyond any medical intervention. Grant and I had driven up to Brisbane when I heard the news that he was very sick. He knew who I was but was in a total delusional state. For whatever reason he chose not to intervene in his own health. I found it challenging to think that such a brilliant mind rejected any form of medical help. He basically denied that there was anything wrong.

Mick's death was incredibly sad. I had spoken to him probably about three weeks before he died, it was during my study at TAFE. He had a condition called drop leg or some such where he lost the strength in his leg. It was painful. He said he missed my cooking and helping. I told him I may be able to get away over the term break.

Upon recollection after Mick's death, it was a conversation where I was left with considerable *"what ifs ..."*

What if I had left my study and moved back there? Could he still be alive?

The world is full of "what ifs" and I can't let these questions affect my life based on information that comes after the fact.

As I said, he died of a preventable disease, which is a tragedy in itself and nothing had prepared me for the phone call from Shane to tell me that Mick had passed away. He was found by one of his yoga friends. He had been dead for a few days and his transition apparently was a slow one. He had collapsed on his patio and not been able to move, taking a few days to die.

Mick was one person who I never thought would die at a relatively early age – in his early 50's. He took his medication sporadically and self-administered his own doses.

I went up for the funeral and wake after and had a few days with Shane and Neil. At the wake there were a lot of people I hadn't seen for a long time. Many of the men who had originally come up to the Northern Rivers to retire due to their diagnosis had gotten better. Medication and lifestyle combined had changed these peoples' lives and so a lot had moved back to the city to pick up where they had left off. I was a bit overwhelmed when men came up to me realising who I was. I was greeted very warmly and with amazement.

'Is that you Greg Kelly? Shit you are a man!' Screamed Steve Mc.

'Last time I looked, Steve: yes, I was.'

There was a gent surrounded by a gaggle of queens who I passed going to the gents. I said: 'How are you?' He looked at me and didn't recognise who I was.

His reply was: 'I can't deal with people at the moment.'

Walking back into the room I saw he was surrounded by the gaggle again. I overheard him being asked when he was moving up to the Northern Rivers and his reply was one that I had heard many times before.

'When I get it together and the time is right.'

I spoke over the group that surrounded him and said: 'Man you said that 15 years ago when I picked you up at the Clunes shop when you first came to stay with Mick. For fuck sake, change your story!'

He looked at me and slowly he recognised who I was.

'Greg – shit, I thought you were dead! Look at you oh man! Let's catch up.'

I said: 'Yeah, sure.' (Maybe I was sounding sarcastic!)

I got compliments on how well I looked that day and I have to say: a big lesson for me was to not feel obliged to return them. Accepting the comments graciously for possibly the first time in my life was challenging. I realised that I hadn't seen a lot of these men for over a decade. Many of the men who had returned to the rat race; the parties, drinking and drug lifestyle actually looked shit house and I didn't feel like lying.

* * *

My tribute to Mick Hannan, who passed away on February 2, 2011

We may have lost a loved one in body but boy do we have memories both individual and shared of a lived life. He wouldn't want tears today. He would want us to party. Mick was an incredibly passionate person.

There was a word he used (that I don't need to share here) if he didn't like something. He would repeat it over and over.

But if he did like something it was "fantastic". He loved people, his yoga, his home and his life. He loved dancing and good times. He gave me this t-shirt, that I'm wearing saying: 'You'll keep this, won't you?; He was cleaning up.

I remember saying: 'Of course, it's Mardi Gras history.'

That history pales into insignificance as it's now part of Mick's history and an individual memory I have of him.

He was very generous to me. For about 18 months I had the pleasure of living at Hazeldene. The gateway with the star on the post!

We had a few conversations about paying rent he refused. So I did a lot of the cooking and cleaning gladly.

One of Mick's hundreds of friends was over and he said to me: 'What's your story? Are you like a houseboy or something?'

Jokingly, I replied: 'Yeah, I'm the houseboy.'

Nothing was mentioned for a few days and we were watching the news and it was a report on the Gulf War (No. 1). Mick had firm opinions on subjects like war and he was telling me them.

The man that was telling our nation the state of conflict so far was a Brigadier of the name Brigadier Michael Hannan. I said: 'Well I'm not just the houseboy, I'm the Brigadiers Houseboy!' We laughed so heartily on that.

So Mick, to me, was – and is – the Brigadier, The Brigadier of Joy.

Brigadier's Houseboy became my business label for different things I have made and sold.

I have a wealth of memories of a vivacious wonderfully eccentric dear friend. I salute you Mick Hannan for living a beautiful life.

FOUR
DEVELOPING MY METHOD

I was 21 and had been given an early release from my apprenticeship. Six months taken off my four years due to my pretty good results. Some of us were lucky to have worked in the kitchens of professional restaurants. I say professional because I've worked in some very unprofessional places, some with more pluses than minuses and vice versa. The bulk of the students came from hospitals, nursing homes and similar places not normally associated with French cuisine or its terminologies. In those days of trade school Escoffier's French cuisine was about all that was taught.

On impulse I decided to book a trip overseas and possibly get a taste of what it was all about. 'I'd like to go to London and Paris, please,' I told the travel agent.

I'm convinced now I appeared quite naïve. She advised me that there were a few other places that I could visit as well if I liked. It was the first time I seriously looked at a world map and it became "real" I suppose. I'd not ever had a desire to travel before or had ever spoken of travel. It was a bit of a spontaneous celebration and England, France, Italy, Switzerland and Greece were to get a visit from me.

Most of the trip went really well. I even had high-tea at one of those legendary hotels (I was horrified a few years later to learn that the same hotel had to have its kitchens closed and rebuilt due to the infestation of critters).

I'd had my bags and some money stolen in Greece and that had limited my funds to fly back to London. The bags I found in Thessaloniki lost property, at the end of one train route. When I got them back they were virtually empty except for my ticket, diary and a few odds and sods.

I went out to have a look at Thessaloniki and within five minutes someone tried to rob me, so I went back to the train station to wait on the platform. A desolate place, somewhat similar to an outback train station; little station, all platform.

After a short while feeling sorry for myself, I heard voices. As they became clearer I heard: 'I think this is the right platform Thel,' in a broad, Australian accent.

As the older couple sat down, I went over to them and as I hadn't spoken to another English speaker for a few weeks, I asked if they were Australians.

'Bloody oath,' said the man whose name escapes me. As we chatted I found out they were on a walking tour. They came from Melbourne and lived in Kew. We spoke of restaurants and places they liked to eat and then I told them I worked at Mietta's Queenscliff Hotel. Thel looked at me and said: 'No....?' Looking incredulous.

It was their favourite place to eat and they went down there on special occasions. She looked at me and said: 'I had the best dessert I've ever eaten there in February. It was a passionfruit sorbet. We were down there for our anniversary.'

Now it was my turn to look blown away because I

showed her my palm and pointed to a scar on my pinkie. 'See this? I cut myself making that sorbet!'

It really was a sort of "God" moment. The randomness that something like that could ever happen to me was quite mind-blowing. When their train arrived for boarding we said our goodbyes and felt like I'd been given a bit of a gift in faith.

With a renewed spirit, I booked the train from Thessaloniki, through (what was) Yugoslavia, to Paris.

At some town in the middle of nowhere, in the middle of the night, your passport was collected by train guards. I wasn't aware this was going to happen and all I knew was being woken by a guard with a revolver in my face saying: 'Passports. Passports.'

I couldn't move for what seemed hours, the American girl next to me turned and said: 'They are taking all our passports. Where is yours?'

Not being able to speak for a bit I pointed to my money belt and she unbuttoned my pants and got the money belt opened. It was handed to the guard who looked at the picture still waving his gun. 'This is not you,' he said in broken English. With the gun, he pointed at the picture and then me – to my hair. 'Different colour,' he snarled in a heavy accent. He then put the gun down by his side, still holding my passport, suggesting that this wasn't me because of the colour difference (it was the 80's and I was going through my Goth phase! That's what we did!). After ten weeks of a European vacation in summer my hair had gone blonde and lost the black entirely.

I have no idea where the words that came out of my mouth came from, but I looked him in the eye and said: 'In Australia, when our mothers die, the eldest son dies his hair black as a sign of respect to honour her.'

He looked at me and said: 'Your mother ... dead?'

'That's why I'm travelling in Europe; to help with the pain.'

He disappeared and came back 20 minutes later with a sandwich and beer, explaining to me (in much better English this time) that I would get my passport back when I reached the border of Italy. The gifts of food and beer I suppose were a sign of a relatively good man who had a conscience. I don't know. Train guards carrying guns always challenged my Australian sensibility.

*　*　*

Passionfruit Sorbet (Machine Version)

1 cup of passionfruit pulp or any type of fruit puree

1 cup of sugar syrup (based on 1-1 sugar and water)

(You can replace half the volume of sugar syrup with champagne for a drier taste)

The juice and zest of 2 lemons

Splash of a spirit

1 egg white

- Combine all ingredients and taste
- It should be a bit strong (as once it's frozen the cold dulls the flavour down) but a good balance of sour sweet and fruit
- Churn in an ice-cream machine
- The spirit will keep the sorbet soft enough to scoop once frozen
- Without a splash the end result can solidify too much and your dessert becomes a rock. This applies to all sorbets and ice-creams.

***

Sorbet (By Hand or Mix-Master)

The meringue methods tend to be best when you want a fruit-based light sorbet and not really appropriate for a boozier sorbet. The meringue will always be a very sweet end result.

3 egg whites
>1 cup sugar
>Juice and zest of 1 lemon
>Approximately 1 cup of fruit puree
>Splash of a spirit

- Beat the whites on high (with a mix master or whisk)
- Slowly add the sugar till it's all dissolved and the meringue peaks. This means that the mixture will stand up when you pull the whisk out
- Once you're satisfied that the meringue is quite firm (at least 5-6 minutes of beating) fold in the puree and lemon juice quickly. As soon as it's combined, taste and check for sweet, acid and flavour balance
- Add lemon and spirit fold through and get into freezer
- This can also be made with an Italian meringue, which is hot thick sugar syrup poured slowly into the beating whites. And follow same directions with fruit and lemon.

I've made all types of spirit based sorbets. Some like gin, grapefruit and mint, vodka and tonic and many other varieties based on the churned recipe. Omitting the fruit puree all together and substituting virtually any flavour based on the guideline. If, for instance, you want to make a champagne sorbet or any alcohol-based dessert, remember: high alcohol content doesn't freeze, so there is a limit to how much booze you put in your mix. At my days in Queenscliff I made quite a few sorbets that, due to how much booze I put in them, never got to the stage of being a sorbet. They could only aspire to ever be a semi-frozen drink. I have to say gin, grapefruit, mint, semi-frozen drink on a hot day in the kitchen was very much appreciated by some of the kitchen staff.

* * *

Melbourne is a classy, fun place even though the weather can be atrocious. However, it got to a point in the late eighties and early nineties that it was starting to become (or was it already?), a violent place to be. The politics of the time were turning conservative. In 1992, Mr. Kennet was swept into power and he was the catalyst that became the nail in the coffin for me to leave.

There was a period from the mid 1980's where I could walk up to the Exchange Hotel on any night of the week and know at least several people in the crowd. Sundays were my favourite. On the other corner from the pub was a launderette, so I would combine a few social drinks with my domestic duties. This could prove to be dangerous; if I had a few too many drinks I would have to go back on Monday morning to see if my laundry was still there. Only once did I lose a favourite pair of jeans. It wasn't long after losing the jeans that the launderette closed down and Sundays just weren't the same. There was a time looming, where nothing would stay the same.

I lived on Punt Road – one of the main roads into Melbourne – in a groovy two-bedroom apartment. It was a block of three and mine was on the top floor. A sometimes-scary friend of mine, Adrian, once called me *'The Duchess Dowager in her Ice Palace'* in reference to the shade of light blue, called ice blue, that I had a chosen to paint the walls.

Generally, I knew my flat-mates really well before they moved in. I had the pleasure of spending quality time with some dear friends who still to this day are just that: true friends.

There was Peter (also nicknamed Pierre) who I had been to secondary school with, Joanne who I'd gone to trade school with, Jeffrey who had been to the same school but was several years younger than me, and Tony, but I didn't know him as I thought I had. The common thread between all of us was we were all shift workers. Socialising was hard as days off never coordinated with each other. One advantage was that you had some time alone, other than sleep time.

Crowds at my favourite pubs started to become noticeably thinner. Just as the names of the living in my address book became scarcer. Normally I could have walked into the pubs and known so many faces. It came to pass that I would go and not know a soul in what seemed to be a very thinning crowd. I started to average attending two or three funerals a week. I began putting lines or crosses through names in my address book. Then, I got into the habit of putting little R.I.P. next to their names. It wasn't long before the simple act of opening the book to find an address became a nightmare.

The Eurythmics came to town, a concert that I would love to have seen. I remember thinking: *'Maybe John, Bryan, and Steve would like to go?'*

About ten people I thought of, that would love to go - were dead. It was definitely a time for a new address book. I went through four address books this way. Needless to say, I missed out on going to concerts for quite a while.

I never felt much like celebrating. I also lost a lot of living peoples' contact details, which was annoying. In maudlin moments fuelled with booze I'd ceremoniously burnt address books to release the spirits (whatever that meant!).

At this time, in the other "non-gay non-HIV world" Melbourne seemed to get nasty. Within a few years there was the Hoddle Street massacre, Queen Street bombing, Turkish consulate bombing, a murder across the road where a man was shot and dragged across Punt Road leaving a trail of blood, the Park Street bomb, Telstra Office bomb (or was that a shooting, or both?), and the slaughter of policemen in Walsh Street.

Most of these events melded into a blur of death and seemed to fit with what was happening in my personal life. It was hard to focus on anything positive. With so much death these outside events seemed to blur into one. It became a question of *'Did that really happen?'* and for a while I would think *'I must have read that'*, as opposed to how close I actually came. Most of these acts were within a few kilometres from me and my home.

Nearly fifteen years or so later, I was in a bar in Adelaide and a gentleman walked up to me and asked if my name was Greg. 'Do you know a guy called Peter and did you live on Punt Road?' He asked me.

'Yes.'

'You don't remember me do you?' he continued, 'My name's Stephen. I came over to your house the night after the bomb in Park Street.'

Suddenly, it seemed as if one hundred years of memory came flooding back. I remembered his gruesome story of a woman being trapped in her second storey apartment. The police had called out to her to jump off the balcony as the bomb had destroyed her exit. She had screamed back: 'I can't, I don't have any legs!' They had been blown off by the bomb.

It was a street that I had walked up and down on my way to work for at least three years. Even if I didn't go to work that way, I still used that street travelling to the city.

I remembered I hadn't long gone to bed when the Turkish consulate blew up. I had walked up Toorak Road after getting the last train home from a visit to Mum and Dad's.

On another occasion I received a phone call late at night for Jeffrey. He got off the phone after some time looking very pale and described that his friend who lived in Walsh Street had been at home at the time of the shootings.

For the above reasons and more, I believe the universe was saying to me to hit the road. I remember that I had been at the bar for an hour or two and decided if I was going to be a stranger it had to be in a strange place. Not my hometown. I decided on a date and networked with friends and connections interstate. I packed up my fabulous little apartment, blessed it for the memory and headed north.

My journey included stops in Sydney, Coffs Harbour, Bangalow and Brisbane. In Bangalow I caught up with John and Jed who ran a local nursery and were friends of Michelle, a girlfriend in Melbourne. They had told me that the pub in Bangalow had a kitchen that needed someone to run it.

Suzanne and I met and became friends several years before leaving Melbourne. We met up in Brisbane after she had left Melbourne six months before. We decided to check Bangalow out and after meeting the landlords of the hotel, we decided to open Sugi's at the Bangalow Hotel. The name was Suzanne's idea that I just went along with. Supposedly, it was a combination of the two of our names. Setting up a restaurant was exciting and we did it with Mum and Dad's financial assistance and all our expertise. John and Jed lent us fabulous palms for the restaurant. My big sister Libby designed our logo for street signs and menu boards. We were off and cooking!

Suzanne decided to leave after about six weeks and I was left to do it by myself. This was an acrimonious split. If this experience were a university degree, it would have cost a heap of money and three years more than the twelve months I was there.

An interesting fact: Suzanne, Tony and Mitchell, who all did rather crappy things were all born on August 14th. They taught me many life lessons about what sort of behaviour I will accept from others. I only know of one other person also born on that day who had none of those attributes that's our gorgeous aunt Norma.

Bangalow is about 17 kilometres from Byron Bay and at the time the highway split the main street in two. Huge semi-trailers would tear up the main street. The busy road never worried me that much.

One day I was being waiter and cook, I was serving meals to a small group of people. I saw out of the dining

START WITH YOUR OWN ONION

room window just how fast a bank robbery could take place.

As I was placing the meals on the table I looked and shouted: 'Duck!' I saw a guy pull a gun out as he went into the bank. Within a minute or two, out they came, speeding off on the way to Casino where I think they were later caught. Word spread through town like wildfire. We had watched whilst crouched under the window sill and it was over in a flash. Meals still hot!

Exciting as it was, I still had to do my washing. So with a full basket of dirty tea-towels and clothes, I proceeded to walk down to the little launderette. When I passed the grocery store smiling to Ken and Marlene who ran it, the policeman of the town came running out trying to get his gun out of his holster. In a stuttering voice, he told me to *'Freeze!'* as he pointed the gun at me.

I dropped my washing basket, raised my arms and said: 'What is the problem officer?'

'An average sized man with a blue jumper was seen robbing the Westpac bank today.'

'Yeah, I know. I watched it! Are you accusing me of robbing the bank?'

Marlene put her head out the doorway and said: 'Glen, what's the problem? This is Greg, from the restaurant!'

'Are you sure, Marlene? He is wearing a blue jumper,' he replied.

'Why would someone who has just robbed a bank walk down the street with their dirty washing only a few hours later?' I asked incredulously, getting upset with a gun pointed at me. 'And we have met before just in case you forgot. We met the night you rode the horse into the main bar.'

'I'm a bit foggy about that night.'

'Funny about that,' was all I could say.

It took a couple of minutes before he put his gun away. Thank God for Marlene. She had to convince him though that I wasn't who he thought I was. Later, he would scare my 17 year old waitress, Liza, in an extraordinary way. She was a bubbly, gorgeous full of life person with a commitment to the fine line of working hard and being a teenager. She literally had a job in almost every shop in the main street at some stage or another and I loved having her. Other than great skills, she knew all the gossip in town! It is not often that I related to a person so much younger than me (it is funny how 17 to 28 years old seems like a great chasm, but 40 to 51 years old doesn't seem that far!).

It was a Friday night, and I had a few diners in the restaurant and the public bar was quite busy. Liza was serving a steak sandwich to a customer when a man on a horse came bursting into the bar. The horse skidded and slipped on the tiled surface. The bar went into an uproar. We all heard. I dropped what I was doing and ran out towards the commotion and saw the horse, not believing what I was seeing.

Liza came over to me and said: 'What a dick!' with an almost nonchalant teenage "seen it all before" attitude. She was concerned that she had dropped the sandwich on the floor. I saw the rider of the horse edge the animal to the bar, he grabbed a six pack from the publican. The crowd had scattered to the edges of the room. He manoeuvred the horse around and it slipped. Another commotion set the punters off and a few men grabbed the horse and helped it and the rider out of the bar. We were so glad the horse survived the ordeal.

Life in Bangalow was a little bit slower than that of Melbourne, but the restaurant kept me occupied. I was a bit of a snob really I had *jus lie* on the menu with the steak. *'What is jus lie?'* became the most asked question I've ever been asked in my life, followed by *'What is p-o-l-e-n-t-a?'* The jus lie became *"homemade stock gravy"* and polenta became *"crushed corn fritter"*.

* * *

A typical menu at Sugi's (The Bangalow Hotel)

21/11/92

Entrées:

Homemade Olive, Herb or Garlic Bread
Homemade Tomato Soup (Soup of the Day)
Avocado Salad Served on Roesti Potato & Tapenade
Homemade Pasta with Herbs, Aioli & Parmesan
Local Asparagus with Hollandaise & a Selection of Shaved Cheeses
Chicken Terrine with Papaya Chutney
Cured Salmon on Blinis
All entrées under $8

Mains:

Scallop Mille Feuille on Bisque Sauce
Malaysian Lamb Curry with Rice
Baked Chicken Breast with a Peach & Spanish Onion Sauce
Rib Eye Fillet with a Semi Dried Tomato Jus & Grilled Parmesan & Basil Polenta
Whole Baby Schnapper with Lemon Dressing & Deep Fried Capers

Fish of the Day – Lemon & Vermouth Beurre Blanc (Ask the Waiter)
Polenta & Vegetable Soufflé Served with a Tomato & Mixed Herb Salsa
Mains $14.50

* * *

I found it amazing that Byron, with its huge vegetarian population, was not so familiar with this wonderful foodstuff. It became a staple on the menu. I would change dishes every day, always including a vegetarian polenta dish.

I had been unfamiliar with so many different types of vegetarians. There were those that ate dairy or even fish and those that were strictly vegan. The hardest to make interesting food for are the no onion or garlic, wheat-free vegan. This stretched my classical training and knowledge.

The versatility of polenta is what I love most about it. Following the instructions on the packet to make the porridge and/or a slice-able slab:

- It can be shaped then baked, fried or grilled
- It can be used as a pizza base instead of dough
- Served as an accompaniment to any meal – from a stew or roast, seafood, game or vegetable dish
- It can even be used as a sort-of pancake and given sweet flavours
- I have even used it in my pasta dough
- I have used polenta pan-fried in olive oil till crispy and added grilled eggplant with roasted skinless capsicum with a wedge of ricotta and some pesto or rough chopped herbs

- It is great with babaganoush and roasted capsicums, with parmesan and sardines, bocconcini and sundried tomatoes
- With roast vegies or left over roast meat with some gravy
- Crisped up into cubes with bacon bits and then tossed through a scrambled egg mix
- Or, when heating the egg mix, simply stir cubes of polenta through adding chopped herbs at the end or used anyway you would use mashed spuds. It is a very versatile ingredient.

Polenta was introduced to me at Queenscliff Hotel many years before by Ivana, who was our pasta maker. Every Tuesday and Thursday were her working days and it was always the day that you would get superb staff meals because they were made by her. The first time she made a polenta dish was similar to a pizza. It was a layer of polenta as a base topped with fresh bocconcini, Western Australian sardines, fresh herbs, semi-dried tomatoes and some parmesan. It was beautiful, elegant and simple. Most of the staff wanted seconds. Unfortunately, there wasn't enough.

Ivana would make anywhere from 15 to 20 kilos of pasta in her two days.

Trays were set on racks which filled large sections of the cool-room. Not only did she roll and cut up trays of tagliatelle and fettuccine, filled pasta dishes were also her speciality. She prepared wonderful ravioli, cannelloni and lasagne with special fillings.

My favourite thing was the cannelloni filling which was a simple mixture of chicken breast, ham, mushrooms, parmesan and freshly grated nutmeg, sautéed together and made into rough forcemeat.

Most mornings when I would come in to work, Ivana had already been working for an hour or two. She would have prepared the fillings for the stuffed pastas and I would scoop some into a fresh baked roll or have it on hot buttered toast.

It would be: 'Bongiorno Mamma. Come stai?'

And she would always respond: 'Bene grazie.'

Once she brought in photos of her and her husband Claudio taken in the 1950's. Both of them appeared to have stepped out of the movie *La Dolce Vita*. I always thought Ivana looked like Sophia Loren. It was a little game I played with her – that Sophia Loren made our pasta!

Long before it had any tendency to be trendy, Ivana had given me an insight into the world of vegetarianism. Not that Ivana was vegetarian, but vegetables, beans and pulses made up a significant portion of her diet.

* * *

Ivana's Pasta

It's the best pasta I've ever had. 10 eggs to a kilo of flour (fine semolina) and some salt.

For green pasta you cook spinach and puree it till a fine paste, adding this to the dough and substituting paste for an egg *or* add spinach powder. For red pasta tomato paste. For black you can use squid ink. Beetroot powder makes an interesting colour.

On the second-last roll of pasta through the machine, lay a sheet on the bench and place herb leaves on half. Fold the other half onto the herbs and put this sheet through for the last roll. Something like continental parsley stretched over a sheet is a great look.

- Pasta making is all in the resting and the rolling
- After the dough is put together it is left to rest for a good hour
- Once you start rolling the dough through the machine, the objective is to get as much flour/semolina into the dough as possible without overdoing the process
- Once it has started it's best not to stop and the dough should "sit" on your fingertips without stretching down your fingers. This means there is enough flour
- Roll several times through the thicker levels and work down to the thinness you desire
- Leave the sheets to dry off most of the moisture. There is a small period of time when the pasta has dried sufficiently to cut then it passes into being too dry. Don't fret if it dries out too much because it can be broken up into pieces and cooked in soups, stews or used for fresh pasta dishes. The French would call this "peasant style". If doing many sheets they need to be covered with tea towels to stop them drying too much. Fettuccine or tagliatelle are great finished dried off on a clothes horse
- Leave to dry on a bench before putting in a container
- This can last for a month or two as long as it is very dry when put in an airtight container or left with just a cloth over it in a dry area. A pillow case works really well.

* * *

Ivana's Cannelloni Filling

This is one recipe that is a bit vague but hopefully in preparing you will be able to understand what I mean. When it comes to the mushrooms in this recipe, you want a similar volume (not weight) of mushrooms to the 300gms of chicken – so what looks to be a similar size to the chicken. You really can't add too much of the mushrooms ham or chicken. It's just a matter of taste.

300gm chicken breasts or boned skinned legs
    Mushrooms – equal volume to chicken
    300gm ham
    Parmesan cheese – a good handful
    Salt and pepper
    Fresh grated nutmeg

- Chop chicken into smallish pieces
- Get a large pan hot with some oil
- Sauté the chicken
- Now add the mushrooms as the chicken starts to brown
- Now add the cubed ham and sauté all
- When cool, remove from the pot and place in a vitamiser. It doesn't need to be pulp, just well-blended
- Taste and season the mix with parmesan and nutmeg. Blend a bit more adjust seasoning and set aside
- Make your béchamel (white sauce) and have a tomato sauce ready. Bottled pasta sauce or tinned is fine
- On the baking dish, add a good tablespoon of oil

and some of the tomato sauce making sure base is a bit sloppy and covered
- Stuff filling into cannelloni tubes (or fold into parcels with cooked flat square sheets of your homemade pasta, approx. size 15x15cm) then line them up in the dish adding tomato on top and then béchamel
- Bake with some foil for 20 minutes, then take the foil off and let it brown up for ½ hour or so (this depends on your oven)
- Fan forced ovens are a lot quicker, if the seal on your crappy oven is buggered then a lot longer!

If you make too much filling, it's great frozen for later use. It's fabulous on fresh bread as a sandwich filling with some cheese and tomato. It can be added to stews, soups to enrich flavour. It can be added to tomato pasta sauce and mixed with fettuccine, tagliatelle or any of the other pastas.

* * *

Spinach and Fetta Filling

The vaguely vegetarian option is the classic spinach and fetta cheese.

- To a bunch of spinach chop an onion, two to three cloves of garlic
- Sauté the onion and garlic
- Add the spinach. You can use silver beet, beetroot leaves, kale (I've put in some cabbage

just to fill it out), you can use frozen spinach as well
- Once the spinach has cooked down I add the cheese to ¼ fetta I add ¾ ricotta. Now it just depends on how cheesy you like things
- Relatively speaking to a bunch of spinach, 500gm cheese
- I also throw in some nutmeg, parmesan, a handful of breadcrumbs or you can use couscous, or some cooked rice
- I add two eggs just to bind it all salt and pepper to taste. This is great cannelloni filling but also my favourite Spanakopita filling wrapped in filo pastry or puff either into triangles or into a big pie.

* * *

My dear friend Emmanuel Stagno, a great cook, intrigued me with stuffing half-cooked, large pasta shells with a ricotta and spinach filling, laying them out on a baking dish lined with tomato pasta sauce. When they had all been filled, more tomato was added on top and some wine to help the pasta shells soften. A large handful of grated parmesan and pecorino cheeses was also added and the dish covered with foil and baked. There was a little bit of fiddling but when I say large I mean small handful size pasta shells, so three to a serve was a good serving.

* * *

Polenta and Vegetable "Soufflé"

START WITH YOUR OWN ONION

- In a pot sauté 1 chopped onion and a couple cloves of garlic
- 1 capsicum chopped
- 2 good sized zucchini
- Couple of sticks of celery
- Set aside when cooked
- Bring 3 cups of milk to the boil (you can use soy, almond, goat, sheep milk or an alternative, water with a splash of wine, tomato soup with a splash of wine, pasta sauce thinned down with wine or stock. Did I say enough you can use wine?)
- Stirring rapidly, add 1 cup of polenta
- Add vegetables
- Stir in 3 yolks, add pepper and salt, you can add cheese at this stage
- Whisk 3 whites and fold them in
- Pour into a greased baking dish
- Bake in a moderate oven for 45 minutes

* * *

I surmised early in the piece that some people educated themselves on the food they were eating and others didn't.

Ingrid was a woman I shared a house with for a while. She was not the most well-researched vegetarian. She lived on dreadfully overcooked vegetables and cheap plain sweet biscuits, constantly complaining of bad migraines, bad periods, and a never-ending list of allergies and rashes.

One day, I wasn't in the best mood, I snapped: 'Love, I'm surprised you aren't dead, knowing the diet you are on.'

'What is wrong with my diet? I am a vegetarian!' Ingrid retorted.

'You boil the living shit out of the veggies you prepare to the point that they would have no nutritional value at all. And, by the way, your biscuits are made with beef tallow which is a crappy butter substitute even worse than margarine.'

The next day she asked me to leave. I agreed that it was for the best.

During my time living with Ingrid, I got involved in community radio. It was here where I met Terri Tompkins or "Mrs. T".

It was the last night of a six-week broadcast, but a few hours before it was turned off for good the local member announced that, for the first time in history, an indefinite extension had been granted by the radio body concerned. We had all prepared for a bit of a wake for the broadcast and suddenly it had become a birth! The first community radio station to transition from trial-run to full-time.

Mrs. T. appeared in an original fifties pleated frock with a matching little jacket, gloves, hat and jewellery, and her lips were a vibrant pink colour. Because she was so immaculately dressed and somewhat flamboyant I always assumed she was actually a *"he"*. I was well and truly wrong! I found out she had a husband and two fabulous children. She never let that get in the way of a good party though, and how she managed to combine her social and working life with her family *and* get along without a driver's licence whilst living in the country always amazed me.

Bay FM had a long wheelchair ramp leading to reception and it was on this ramp where she and I danced. I loved swinging her and doing a bit of a jive because her frock went off when she twirled.

Arriving at the party she told a story of what had just happened to her at *The Rails* (a Byron pub). Her outfit intrigued one of the punters so much that he asked if he could take a few photos of her and his car. She went to the car park to find a 1950's Thunderbird, the same powdery blue colour as her outfit. So (naturally) she jumped onto the bonnet and away he snapped.

Although a great cook, superb entertainer and hostess, she was also a marvellous guest. Sometimes when different groups of people congregate for events there can be awkward moments when people are starting to mix. This was never a concern when Mrs. T was around. On many occasions I saw a gathering of a few people become a feast and a night for memories. Her vibrancy is infectious and is a beautiful thing.

* * *

Thai-Inspired Red Curry

The sauce for this recipe is delicious and can be used with just about any meat or seafood. With the omission of the prawn paste (belachan), it is a perfect sauce that can be used for a vegan vegetable, bean or tofu curry as well.

1 large chopped onion
1 stick of lemon grass
Equal amounts of galangal and ginger – approximately a tablespoon of each
4-6 curry leaves
2-3 fresh or dried lime leaves
½ tablespoon of prawn paste
1 bunch of coriander roots – cut the bunch generally below the band that keeps the bunch together. Wash them thoroughly and let dry

6 cardoman pods, bruised (give them a squash with the flat side of your knife to help release the flavours)

I use as much as desired with chilli. For a little bite 1 birds-eye should be enough – when it comes to chilli I generally serve what I like and if people want more chilli then serve a small side dish of freshly chopped or some sambal

½ a tablespoon of tamarind paste dissolved in some hot water

6 cloves of chopped garlic *or* 6 heaped teaspoons from a jar

½ tablespoon of sesame oil

2 tablespoons of peanut or vegetable oil

2 cans of coconut cream

2 tablespoons of tomato paste

- Chop and sauté onions in the peanut oil
- Pound ginger and galangal in a mortar and pestle
- Add garlic
- Add to the sautéing onions;
- Prawn paste
- Cardoman pods, slightly crushed, then chilli
- Tomato paste
- Coconut milk
- Leaves, bruised
- Lemon grass, left whole to be easily removed after cooking
- Tamarind to taste.
- Cook the mixture till it has reached a flavour balance

- Take out the lemon grass and let the mixture cool.
- Puree the mixture and strain
- Bring to the boil and taste.

Alternative method:

- Sauté the onions
- Throw in whole cloves of garlic, smallish knobs of ginger and galangal, prawn paste, cardoman pods, then the rest
- Cook up and bring to the boil
- Let cool for a while and then puree the ingredients, then put through a fine strainer
- Bring to boil and taste.

For both methods:

- Once it has been re-boiled, check for salt, sweet, tang from tamarind, and full mouth flavour
- Then this sauce is added to the meat or vegetables
- It can be used in a crock pot, on the stove, or used in a roasting tray with meat or vegetables
- When it's finished, add some lime and salt to taste if needed.

This is a great sauce that can be prepared ahead a day or two before being used. It's a good thing to put some into the freezer to use on another day.

*** * * ***

Annesley's Chicken Korma
    1 kg chicken
    45gm cadjanuts (cashews)
    5-6 sprigs of coriander
    2 sprigs parsley
    ½ inch stick cinnamon
    60gm onion
    2 cloves
    250gm plain yoghurt
    1-2 teaspoons lime juice
    1 tomato
    30gm coconut
    1 dessertspoon coriander ground
    2 green chillies *or* 2 teaspoons of chilli powder
    3 cloves garlic
    1 ½ teaspoons salt
    Slice of ginger
    3 cardoman pods
    3 dessertspoons of vegetable oil

The one thing that I learnt when making the same curry many times is that they can be all different!

- The method for this dish is to sauté the onions and spices together
- Either in the same large pot or a large oven dish

add the chicken, making sure all the meat is covered in the spices
- And the yoghurt and stir through
- If baking in the oven, cover with foil and bake for at least an hour in a moderate oven
- If cooking on a stove, bring the mixture to a boil with the lid on then turn it down as low as possible and cook for at least an hour. This is the least preferable way to do it
- This can also be done in a crock pot and I have to say: during winter, putting this on in the morning and coming home to a Korma crock pot is divine
- This can also be a great sauce for vegans by omitting the yoghurt and substituting for a vegetable stock, soy yoghurt or any vegetable liquid

* * *

Annesley's Burryiani

750gm lean lamb, cubed
3 dried chillies
½ cup hot water
6-8 cloves of garlic
1 tablespoon of fresh ginger
2 tablespoons fresh coconut, grated
2 tablespoons blanched almonds
1 tablespoon ground coriander
1 teaspoon of ground cumin
1 teaspoon poppy seeds
½ teaspoon of ground fennel
½ teaspoon of ground cardoman

¼ teaspoon of ground cloves
¼ teaspoon of ground mace
½ teaspoon of black pepper
4 tablespoons of ghee (or oil)
1 medium onion chopped
4 cardoman pods bruised
½ teaspoon of ground turmeric
½ cup yoghurt
2 tomatoes peeled and chopped (or 1 small tin)
1 ½ teaspoons salt
1 teaspoon of garam marsala
2 tablespoon of chopped fresh coriander

- Soak chillies in water for 5 to 10 minutes
- Under a griller or in the oven, toast the garlic, ginger and coconut for a few minutes
- Add these to a blender with the almonds, chillies and water
- Toast the ground coriander, cumin, poppy seeds and fennel then add to blender
- Then add cardoman, cloves, mace and pepper
- Sauté onions, cardoman pods, turmeric and the blended ingredients
- Add yoghurt and tomatoes last and get off the heat
- Sprinkle the salt onto meat and then coat the meat with the sauce
- Bake in a closed casserole until meat tender for approximately 1 ½ hours in a moderate oven.

* * *

Pickled Sprouts

START WITH YOUR OWN ONION

For about a dollar a bag at the market, these are a great accompaniment to a curry. If the curry is a bit hot these can cool it down a bit.

Sprouts
Vinegar
White wine
Sugar
Ginger
And a little julienne of carrot

- Put the sprouts in a colander and give them a quick wash
- Put into a jar or container and you need enough liquid to fill the jar
- Equal parts of vinegar and wine with sugar to taste
- For every cup of liquid, a good teaspoon of ginger and maybe a heaped soup spoon of sugar
- Bring liquids to a boil and then add sugar – don't add it all at once, maybe divide into 3 lots and taste it as you go
- The ginger and carrot are added and taste should be a pleasant combination of acid sweet and ginger
- When cool, pour onto sprouts in the jar
- This should be stored in the refrigerator
- Its lovely served with red meaty things, spicy curry dishes, in a salad with an Asian flavour, or sprinkled in cold rolls.

* * *

Cous-Cous

When making cous-cous, it's by far the easiest and quickest carb, use orange juice with some cinnamon stick instead of water. At the end of the cooking process add a good knob of butter to loosen it all up. Some preserved lemon chopped up is also lovely through it.

* * *

Rissoles – Chicken, Beef, Lamb, Kangaroo

500gm mincemeat (any)
¾ cup of breadcrumbs
1 cup milk
2 teaspoons of garlic
Salt and pepper
1 egg
If you're making a lot of burgers the ratio is generally mincemeat 1 to 1/3 bread crumbs

- Soak bread crumbs in warm milk – add enough milk so the crumbs come together and aren't sloppy but not too firm either
- When cool, add to the meat
- Next the egg, garlic, salt and pepper
- At this stage you can also add some chopped onions, roasted garlic, a tablespoon of mustard, chopped herbs
- Also some things I've added: a few tablespoons of chutney, Worcestershire sauce, sweet chilli sauce, any condiment that you can find. I tend to go through the cupboards and refrigerator

and look for bits and pieces that need to be used up
- This mixture can be rolled into small or large meat balls or rolled up in puff pastry and make sausage rolls out of
- Or bake it all together and make a meat loaf.

FIVE

DRESSING THE LAYERS

Schooling, 1970-1981

I attempted to end my life when I was about fourteen years old. I had stolen a few of Mum's Valium and was sitting in the kitchen preparing myself to swallow them. I had been in the house alone for a few hours and thought I had some more time – until I heard the lock click in the front door. It was Mum. She looked at me suspiciously and asked me if I was all right. I said I was and went outside putting the pills into my pocket.

Sitting out on the brick wall underneath a huge rhododendron tree (my favourite place to think), thinking about what might have happened if I *had* done the deed and Mum had walked in to find me dead. I hadn't thought about the ramifications of anyone finding my body and realised then that it wouldn't be the nicest thing to do to anyone else.

I kept the pills in a little plastic container for a few years – more as a symbol than anything else. Those little white pills had a certain mystique about them. I could stare at them for hours going over in my head *'could I do it?'*.

I look back on this period with a certain amount of

START WITH YOUR OWN ONION

dread. I hated going to school; there wasn't a day that went by I wasn't picked on, punched or abused.

It was the second term of Third Form and even the teachers where getting in on the act. I had walked into the science room and the class was laughing hysterically and they all turned and looked at me. Wadi, the science teacher, ran across the other side of the classroom to his overhead projector and grabbed the sheet that was on it. It was too late for him to cover up his deed though. He had written, projected up onto the wall, Greg Kelly has a chicken's arsehole.

I sat in that room listening to the chant that was ringing in my head. It took ages for it all to subside. In fact, there were only a few minutes of actual lesson. The rest of the time was spent trying to control the chants of *"chicken's arsehole"* over and over from the boys, starting as a low murmur, building to a crescendo and starting all over again. I confronted the teacher after class and asked him if he had actually written what I thought he had and he said: 'Well, haven't you?'

These were not the days of students being able to sue teachers for improper conduct. These were the days of the bully, and because I had no desire to pick on anyone, I was the one being picked on. Maybe it was because the only role I knew how to play in this jungle was the victim. I was a child who really didn't think I had much in the way of coping skills. Support from teachers was mixed with *'It will strengthen his character'* or *'Well that's what he is, so he deserves it.'*

What I learned from religious schooling was if you were different – and let's face it: I was a Nancy boy – Jesus was on the bully's side. Because if you weren't masculine enough, you deserved punishment.

There was another time when Mum had come up to the school to see the Form Coordinator to complain about the amount of times that she had to mend my uniforms and the amount of bruises I was receiving. The next day the teacher concerned came into the classroom and wanted to know who was picking on Greg Kelly for being a poofter. He commanded that everyone concerned stand up on the platform. Of forty students, one other kid and I were still seated. The teacher called in a few more teachers and everyone was given six straps each. I felt like I was the most hated human being on the planet in that moment. The persecution went to a whole new level. It went from just *most* people thinking I was a lowlife to *everyone* hating me.

Pat Benatar sang '*Love Is a Battlefield.*' I thought that was crap; school was the battlefield and after everyone had been punished, war was declared on me.

During this time, I remember trying to exit the classroom one day as soon as the teacher had left at the end of the period. Before I could, I was dragged on the floor back into the classroom by all the boys, spat at, punched, screamed at and verbally abused. I remember I was wearing ugg boots that had leather straps (it was casual dress day). They pulled the straps off my boots and hit me with them.

One of the major issues I remember dealing with when I came out, after leaving school and coming to terms with my sexuality, was that all those mother-fucking arse-wipes were right; I am a poofter. Instead of the dirty poofter that they called me for twelve years of my life, I had to figure out what a "good" poofter was.

How I survived the whole experience of school still baffles me. I passed most of the exams with the exception of a couple of semesters when the only thing I thought about was exiting this planet. Now in my fifties, I believe it was a huge lesson in life that has made me the better person (the further I get away from my youth the better, though).

* * *

I only truly started to live when I finally left school and went out into the real world. Many years later, during a visit to Mum and Dad, I remember being at Brandon Park (a shopping centre) for some reason. I had entered the complex and within a few seconds I heard my name being called. I turned and saw that it was Grant; the ring leader of the bullies – the arsehole that had made my life hell. I said hello and he greeted me as if we were long lost friends, seemingly very happy to see me. I asked what he was up to and I found out that he'd had about 15 jobs since leaving school and hadn't done much with himself.

All the protection given to him (he was a swimming star who could do no wrong) from the priests and this is where he got! I have to say, I relished in telling him I had been chosen for an apprentice of the year competition, that I had bought a car, I was planning a trip overseas and was quite happy with myself. I said farewell and as I walked away, for the first time ever, I really felt (for a second in time) I was a winner.

* * *

1996

The suppressed issues I had with bullying started to present years later when I was diagnosed with a type of pneumonia (PCP) common with people who have HIV. I started having violent dreams about blowing up kids in the quadrangle. My therapy was to write it down and get it out;

to exorcise the demons. It did help, but one thing it wasn't helping was the fact that my weight had gone from 69 kilograms to 49 in about a month.

I walked into my doctor's office one day pulling down my pants and grabbing the sagging flesh from my arse and saying: 'Look at this Paul. This is not good. My arse looks like Endora's face and I'm too young to have starred in Bewitched.'

I could literally pull the skin from my bum half way up my back. It was definitely not a good look. I was really starting to freak out. The new medication I was on was giving me this side-effect. My wonderful doctor, Paul, who (along with many others) is one of the reasons I am still alive, suggested I go on a high-fat diet. To some, going on a high-fat diet might mean a bit more cream and ice cream with dessert. To me, it was mixed grills smothered in hollandaise sauce followed by huge bowls of ice cream and chocolate sauce.

Rapid weight loss is a very scary thing to go through. My once reasonable frame had morphed to ugly before my very eyes. The stretchy skin and muscle wastage resembled horror movie makeup. My cheeks sunk into my face and flesh hung from my bones with no tone to it. It wasn't *me* I was looking at in the mirror each morning. I looked and felt like I was going to die and I didn't want to go – not like this, anyway. I prayed for a bus or car (preferably a Silver Cloud Rolls Royce) speeding down the highway to help me onto glory ...

Although I looked like shit, I really didn't want to die. There were a few things that I did to turn the tide around. My high-fat diet made me pay more attention to what I was eating in a different way than I normally would. I despised the tubs of yoghurt or anything that proudly proclaimed "low-fat" and looked long and hard for everything that was high in fat.

For about three months I had mixed grill for lunch every day. Lamb chops, sausages, rissoles, bacon, bread fried in butter and eggs. I don't think I could ever do another mixed grill, but it achieved the result I wanted. I walked around very proud of my little belly.

The other thing that I took up in earnest was rehydration fluid. This was way before the variety of sport drinks available today (which I wouldn't go near. Far too many colours). To make it, I'd dissolve four Chlorvescent tablets, six teaspoons of sugar and one teaspoon of sea-salt in a cup of boiling water then add two litres of water. When this was recommended to me the science behind it seemed quite simple. The body normally doesn't absorb all the plain water you drink, but with the dissolved sugar and salt your body grabs these molecules that have water molecules attached to them. As I was having so much diarrhea and vomiting I was losing too much fluid from my body. This liquid was to help replace the fluid lost.

My girlfriends were the first to notice the change in me. I kept getting comments about the clarity of my eyes and smoothness of my skin. I was very proud that I had brought myself back from death's almighty embrace. To be at the point where I thought *this is it* and then come back has made me appreciate life so much more. It's an experience that I wouldn't wish on anyone (unless they had a death wish). I was happy, but angry that life was being taken away from me over a long, slow, protracted period.

* * *

In Melbourne, in my Punt Road days, a friend of mine tried

to "do the deed" (attempt suicide). Tony was a friend and flatmate who had a heroin addiction. I was very naïve in thinking he could give it up just like giving up lollies for Lent or coffee – something benign. I had no capacity or reference point for what addiction was. I wasn't aware of the grip it could take on your soul until Tony slashed his wrists so many times there was nothing for the doctors to stitch up. He had to have some sort of pig skin layered around his wrists for them to heal. For the amount of slash marks he had given himself, each one had missed the one vein he needed to get to achieve the aim of the exercise.

I will never forget when he came back to the flat with bandaged wrists very down trodden and weak. I couldn't comprehend that someone I knew could be so brutal to themselves. It was the most horrendous thing I had ever seen up to that point in my life. I asked him, if he wanted to end his life, why hadn't he just used heroin. His reply disturbed me – he said because he was so used to it, it would probably cost over two thousand dollars to do that.

He was one of the reasons why I had to start believing in a greater power. Not because of what he had done, but how it happened. He tried to take his life on the banks of the Yarra River late one night in August. This particular night happened to be a warm, humid night – something not normal in Melbourne. Because of the humidity, his blood clotted and congealed around the slash marks, thus saving his life.

* * *

Another time in Kin-Kin (Queensland) in the late 90's I was left to look after a friend's property that his parents had given him. Shaun was a middle-aged artist – a brilliant one at that. He had a much younger lover, Marcel. Marcel was a beautiful young man who seemed to have everything going for him. The boys had parted at this time and whilst Shaun was away, Marcel came up for a few days to chill out. I had a soft spot for Marcel, and because they weren't together I thought I might have a chance!

On the last day we were alone before Shaun came back from his holiday I had been at Robbie's place all day helping her in her garden. I drove into the driveway that evening and parked the car full of excitement. I could hear the stereo blaring out some heavy-duty techno music and smiled to myself that he must be a little bit drunk. When I got to the house I saw him dancing in an "out of it" way, with one arm wrapped in a towel. I walked in and as he hugged me I saw the towel soaked in blood ...

'Oh Greg, it is so good to see you,' he slobbered.

'What has happened?' I asked, realising his blood was running down my back.

'I was making dinner and your knives are so beautiful and sharp. I just wanted to see what would happen.'

I felt like punching him. Any thoughts of an intimate night flew out the window as I administered some basic first aid. My first thought was to call an ambulance and get him to a hospital. I went to pick up the phone and he refused to let me call anyone.

'No! They will keep me in for days! I'll be committed! No, you can't!' He was adamant and I realised in that moment he had done this before – he knew the system.

I turned the stereo off and looked at him and said: 'Let me look at what you've done or I am leaving and will call the police.' He let me look at the wounds he'd made. They were about six slashes 10 to 15 centimetres long.

'Fuck, why?' I said.

'It feels good,' he whispered.

I cleaned the wounds, found a first aid kit and bandaged them. He kept waving his arms around trying to dance and kept saying everything was okay – that he loved doing it and he knew what he was doing. I sent him to bed with a threat of still calling someone if he didn't go and it didn't take long before he was asleep. I looked at the house which had been trashed with blood spots here and there and then I went into the kitchen – where the deed had been done. Blood was on most of the benchtop and down the sides of the doors. The brutality of what I was looking at is still hard to conceive. It resembled a movie set; appearing almost fake. Unfortunately, this was no made-up scene. I cried for a moment and started to clean the mess – there was no way I would have been able to deal with it in the morning.

My attention turned to the sink and realised he had done this horrible deed with *my* knives. On many occasions I have thrown all of my knives into a sink full of soapy water and washed them without ever getting cut. This time as I was cleaning them, my knives bit me from the sink twice in a matter of seconds. I remember thinking they (my knives) were really pissed at being treated this way. I had to get advice on how to release the bad energy from my knives because if I didn't I knew they would be useless. What do you do with something so precious that has been used in such an insidious way? I loved my knives, they were an extension of my hands.

My dear friend Robyn told me to place them in an earthenware dish with rainwater and some crystals under the next full moon. I did as I was directed and they have never bitten me since.

Both Shaun and Marcel had a long history with heroin and Shaun told me that he attributed their giving up to me.

I'm not sure if I believe him, but it would be nice to think I am that powerful. As far as I'm concerned, he did the work.

I went around one night to their place after trying for about a week to contact them. I bashed on the door for a while to get their attention. Unbeknownst to me, they thought it was the police so they tried to hide everything. I had brought with me a beautiful charcoal drawing Shaun had done for me of Kings Beach. I put it under his face and demanded he sign it.

'What's the hurry? I'll do it in a moment,' he said.

I screamed at him: 'If you are going to do a Brett Whitely on me – and it is pretty obvious you are going to – I want you to sign this now. This will be my pension fund with your signature. Without it, it won't be worth anything."

＊＊

Dressings

Vinaigrette

Vinaigrette is the simplest of quick dressings. I have never found it better to buy already prepared varieties.

- The standard generally is a combination of one third acid to two thirds of oil
- This now depends on your taste – you can easy add a bit more or less of any ingredient
- Mustard, garlic, chopped herbs, spring onions, salt, pepper can all be added to taste
- This will last a long time when stored in the fridge and will just get better over time
- You can add a tablespoon of mustard to a cup of

vinaigrette and put it all in a blender with the end result being a sort of mayonnaise
- An interesting thing to add to a dressing can be blue cheese with a bit of brandy and cream. Squash the cheese and combine with the liquids. This is a strong dressing that would need to go with equally strong flavours – good on roasted veggies.

* * *

Ginger and Sesame Dressing

1 ½ tablespoons grated fresh ginger
3 shallots minced or 3 spring onions chopped fine
½ cup rice wine vinegar
2 limes
2 tablespoons soy sauce
1 scant tablespoon sesame oil
1 cup olive or peanut oil
1/3 cup toasted sesame seeds
½ bunch chopped coriander
Salt and pepper to taste

- Blitz ingredients together to form a smooth dressing, then season
- This is a great dressing that can be used on cold meat platters. When it's warmed and combined with hot blanched vegetables, it makes a great salad dressing or goes well with barbequed chicken or fish
- To season the end result there are a few options I like:
- You can add a good splash of fish sauce, sherry

or freshly toasted and ground coriander seeds to taste
- A tablespoon in a fish, veggie or chicken broth with some steamed rice is good as a quick satisfying meal.

* * *

A Bit of a Tartare Dressing
1 tablespoon Capers
1 tablespoon Cornichons
1 onion, finely chopped (I like to sweat the onions separately in a pan with a little oil and then add them to the dressing as raw onions has a tendency to give me gas!)
¼ bunch chives
1 lemon juice
1 tablespoon parsley, chopped
6 spring onions, chopped
A little thyme, chopped
A few rosemary leaves

- You can chop all the ingredients separately and combine or you can put all ingredients in a blender and puree then season to taste
- Again, this is a versatile dressing that can be used on most things, but is really good with cooked fillets of fish.

* * *

Asian-Inspired Dressing

This is a great sauce for all sorts of meats and tofu. It's great for fresh, steamed or roasted vegetable salads and a fabulous sauce for a cold lamb salad or on steamed veggies.

> 2 birds eye chillies (if chilli isn't your thing ½ a chilli will give it some zing but not freak out taste buds)
> 1 medium sized onion, chopped
> 6 curry leaves
> Good knob of galangal – this is about the size of half an adult thumb
> Same size of ginger
> Sesame oil to taste
> Dessertspoon of hoi sin
> 1 tablespoon of soy sauce
> 2 cups chicken stock

- Make a paste in a mortar and pestle with dry ingredients or blitz in a machine
- When you think it's enough pounding and you've gotten some frustration out of your system, sauté the paste in a little oil
- Then add stock and sauces. Reduce by half
- You could be forgiven if you didn't have a lot of time to sauté roughly chopped ingredients and brown well
- Add the stocks and sauces and, when reduced, strain the liquid
- Cool and serve on salad or rice on meat etc.

* * *

Mango Sauce
2 mangoes, pureed
¾ cup of mayonnaise
¾ cup of whipped cream
1 large lemon or 2 limes, juiced (but you could also add the equivalent of any citrus that had some good tartness to it).

- Combine all the ingredients together with only ½ whipped cream at first, then fold in rest
- Season according to taste
- Serve with cold seafood or seafood salad.

* * *

Great Marinade for Red Meat
This is good for a stir fry or thin cuts of meat, or can be used for cooking ribs, baking and slow cooking. (This can obviously be cut down and made according to taste)

4 tablespoons peanut or vegetable oil
4 tablespoons of soy sauce
2 tablespoons of honey
2 tablespoons of vinegar
1 teaspoon of ground aniseed
4 cloves of garlic
1 teaspoon ginger (fresh or ground)

- Combine all ingredients together, mixing thoroughly
- If you are making a stir fry there's not really any need to marinate the meat for any period of

time because it's a quick meal. So the meat can be tossed through with some of the dressing and cooked straight away
- If you are baking ribs, you can coat the meat and let to marinate over a period of time. Overnight if you desire, but at least a few hours before cooking.

* * *

Beurre Blanc for Two
50gm unsalted butter
½ cup stock
¼ cup cream
1 dessertspoon of vinegar or wine

- Bring wine and vinegar to a boil and add stock
- Reduce further by half and add cream
- When it's nice and thick and about the consistency of runny cream, add knobs of butter and whisk over heat. The butter will thicken the sauce
- To finish you can add some chopped herbs just before serving.

A simple version of this can be made when you have:

- Pan fried your chicken fish or steak
- Set the meat aside and add some stock, wine or water to pan

- Let it boil and grab all the lovely caramelised bits from the pan
- When this is boiling, add some cream about a tablespoon, and let reduce then add butter to thicken the sauce
- Be aware, if you are cooking for two or four people then you are dealing with small amounts – so probably no more than a cup of liquid depending on the size of what you are cooking in. Probably ½ cup liquid for two people of sauce
- When making a pan sauce, you can also add the liquid and reduce, omit the cream and just thicken the pan juices with knobs of butter.

* * *

Oysters San Francisco

San Francisco Cream 1970's style menu at the Melbourne Oyster Bar

I have popped this one out at parties and some love it because it's retro, others because it's decadent and some people love it because they love rich food! If anything, these oysters are showy!

1 cup of sour cream
2 tablespoons of finely chopped prawn, crab or cray meat
½ chopped medium onion
1 tablespoon of chopped dill

1 tablespoon of spring onions
2 lemons, juiced and zests
1 jar of whatever fish roe you like (the black lump-fish roe or the salmon roe is good)

- Mix all together (except caviar and cray meat)
- Put teaspoons on to oysters and then small dollops of meat and roe
- Depending on the people and the party they can be an extravagance, but also a bit of fun if retro is your thing!

* * *

A Vague Curry Sauce

Onions

Garlic and an equal amount of ginger

Butter, ghee or oil used to cook the onions

Curry powder (this is really depending on taste. There are lots of powders out there. I always urge to under estimate than overdo it. You can always add flavour but it's hard to take it out!)

Coconut milk

Seafood or chicken stock or water

- Always start with sautéing onions, garlic, then spices (in this case, the preferred curry powder)
- Add the coconut milk or cream
- Now add stock and cook till it's a good consistency
- If you are having a meat curry, it can be coated

in half the curry powder, sealed and browned and added to the sauce
- Place it in a baking dish in the oven and cook till tender (or you'll get a great result in a slow cooker)
- If you are making a seafood curry, it's best to add the raw seafood to the hot finished sauce and cook the seafood that way
- This sauce can be poured over browned meat or raw seafood put in a tray, covered with foil and baked in the oven or on top of the stove
- Run out of oil? Couldn't be bothered going to the shop but have everything else? If you don't shake the tin of coconut milk or cream beforehand, scoop the thick top off. This can be used to sauté onions with the top layer (¼ of the can)
- To cut a curry's bite, add fresh tomatoes, coconut or potatoes to the sauce

* * *

Thai Beef Salad Dressing

This is one of my favourites for taste and versatility.

1 bunch of spring onions
1 bunch each of coriander and mint
4 cloves of garlic
4 chillies
120ml soy sauce
80ml lemon juice
30-40ml fish sauce

Sugar to taste (about a teaspoon)

- Blitz it all together or combine by hand
- You can add 1 can coconut milk to recipe
- And lime juice and zest.

* * *

Herb Paste

For just about anything. This paste is great with steamed or fresh oysters. It's so flexible. A dessertspoon into a broth with some rice or potatoes, or as a dressing for cold meat or salad.

3 cloves of garlic
Same amount of ginger
6 roughly chopped spring onions
Chilli, salt and pepper
Juice and zest of a large lemon
1 teaspoon of sesame oil

- Add ingredient into the mortar and pestle
- Blend till fine
- Season accordingly
- I have this keep in the fridge for weeks. It gets better with a little time.

* * *

Crème Anglaise

1 litre of milk
100gm sugar

10 yolks

Split vanilla pod (or small splash of a brandy or other spirit or liqueur instead of imitation vanilla)

- Warm milk and separately combine yolks and sugar
- Add whisked yolks and sugar to the milk and heat – but not to the boil
- Keep stirring. This can be done on the stove, in a bowl on a pot, with water as well. Just be aware not to boil the water. You will end up cooking the egg yolks and your sauce is a bit buggered!
- Anglaise is ready when it coats the back of the spoon. If it looks like it might be too hot, best to pour it onto a flat tray with sides to cool rapidly
- Place in fridge or freezer for a few minutes to cool down fast.

* * *

Crème Patisserie (thick custard)

12 yolks
450gm sugar
75gm flour
25gm cornflour
1.2 litres of milk
Vanilla

- Heat milk
- Add yolks, sugar and flours together
- Add to heated milk
- Stir well

- It's best to cook this in a bowl that's big enough to be placed over a pot of water and let the steam cook it. It needs to be stirred or whisked to stop it from forming lumps, but you can put the whole thing in a food processor (once cooked) if it does get lumpy. Cooking over a pot like this stops it from sticking and burning.

SIX
REPEAT THE BASICS

It never ceases to amaze me how people in their active addictions can somehow win the lotto or put a 20 cent piece into a machine and win a stash of money. They may owe heaps to friends and family, but generally there's a shifted priority. I've seen a trusted friend and flatmate steal the rent money, ransack the apartment, and spray paint *AIDS poofter, cunt* on the walls of my lounge room for his habit.

Another character, her name was Hazel – an interesting Queensland identity, who came to stay for a few days when Shane and I were sharing a unit in Byron was given $20 by her girlfriend to go and play golf. Instead of playing golf, she put the money into a slot machine, won a couple of grand and proceeded to drink for the rest of the day. She came back to our place that evening well and truly plastered, empty of cash and collapsed on the couch for the evening. Unfortunately, she didn't make it to the toilet that night. I gave the job of cleaning the couch to Shane. This was a priceless moment that we have both laughed at till we had tears rolling down our faces! *'She came, she drank, and she pissed on the couch!'*

Then there was Shaun, who went into thirds with two other friends in the lotto. The ticket won, Shaun picked up the money and it mysteriously disappeared.

It appears to me when someone needs a thousand dollars more for heroin, that money can just appear. Tony, Hazel and Shaun should all be dead – but they aren't (as far as I am aware at the time of writing). I should be dead – but I'm not. Why can't people seem to manifest money when they are straight in the same way as when they are on their chosen poison?

I may or may not have had an addiction to pot. I would suggest that side effect of vomiting for many years has led to a bit of a dependency on it, but I can – and have – gone without it for months on end. I do think the use of pot has helped more than it has hindered me – especially when it comes to eating. The medication over the last few years has been much better than it was in the past (I only have side effects like heart attacks now, as opposed to daily vomiting and bouts of diarrhea 20 to 30 times a day).

I recently have come through the other side of a particularly nasty chest infection which coincided with my carpets being changed. For whatever reason, the dust on top of the infection irritated my lungs and immune system and I started to have night sweats and they triggered flashbacks to nights gone by. Horrible as they are, I seemed to know what to do almost unconsciously. I remember the first night they reoccurred: I awoke about 4am drenched in sweat. I lay there until it got too unbearable. I had a quick shower, stripped the bed sheets, put new ones on and lay out a fresh towel on the other side of the bed where I slept. I then slept till about 8am and awoke drenched again. I got up and started washing sheets and towels. This became a pattern for about 10 days. I went to the doctor and told her about the sweats and other symptoms. She mentioned that they had a sort of post-traumatic connection. I said to her that usually if I am sick it's because of HIV medication side effects, and it was interesting getting a sickness that "normal" people got. I felt too healthy within myself to have HIV-related pneumonia.

I believe that in being part of the HIV community during the eighties and nineties, having my own HIV-related illnesses, caring for friends who died, going to over 80 funerals – it felt like a war, and I had nagging survivors guilt .

It's weird how night sweats triggered so many issues from my past that I thought I had laid to rest. I had dreams of dying, of being useless and valueless.

2003

I did a short presentation on HIV/AIDS and PTSD and a follow up essay at TAFE for a Certificate III in Community Welfare. I felt brave doing this, thinking that the whole confidential thing would be respected. A few days after the presentation, I was in the library and a woman who had her own issues with alcohol came up to me and said in a loud voice: 'Greg! Shit, man! I didn't know you had AIDS! That's shit, man. I suppose you're gonna die soon. Shit! I couldn't believe when I found out you got AIDS.'

I looked around to see about 30 peoples' mouths wide open. She seemed oblivious to this though, and continued in a *blah, blah, blah* sort of way. I remember I said: 'I don't have AIDS – I'm HIV positive,' and walked out of the library.

I had to get to the bus stop, which wasn't very far, but it

suddenly felt as far as a large football field. It became the school quadrangle where I was belted up and abused. It became a rather harrowing place – a place of fear. The little abused boy seemed to take over in my head. It was getting late, a bit before twilight, which made it even worse. I hated that bitch.

I realised she had, with her large mouth, taken away a certain freedom and bravado I thought I had possessed. I felt the energy that kept my feet on the ground slipping away from me. My self-protection was already pretty flimsy, and I felt like a bullied school kid again. I got on the bus. No one followed. No one bashed me, but they had in the past – and I remembered that.

This episode unfolded in the last few weeks of the school year. I asked the lecturer before the next class if I could have some of the class time. I told her what had happened in the library and she gave me the time I needed. I had to speak for the clients, who these students would be working with in the future. I felt victimised by whomever and whatever had hurt me. Whoever had broken my confidentiality needed to know how it felt. I got in front of the class and explained what had happened in the library, almost raised my voice, and asked: 'How fucking dare one of you take away my freedom like that? If this was the real world, and I was a client, you wouldn't be going to a nice comfortable home tonight, because I would have taken it from you. I have the opportunity to sue your arse off. How could anyone gossip about this?'

There were tears from a lot of the students. I was glad I had made a bit of an impact. I made sure I looked everyone in the eyes. They all were going to see my fear and rage. A few days later, two young women, 17 or 18 years old, came up to me and apologised. They told me they had been talking about me and the woman in the library had overheard them. I thanked them, but reminded them that I still would have their houses in the real world.

Debriefing is a very important thing to do in the community welfare sector (and in the wider world), especially dealing with clients issues. It is also vital to remember to close the door or at least make sure there is NO ONE within ear shot.

* * *

For the following paper, I have taken bits and pieces of research from the internet. I must acknowledge I am remiss at acknowledgements. The demands and level of this course were okay, but not high. At this stage I was very unaware of writing essays and protocols of such. Accrediting was a higher skill expected at Diploma level, so expectations were at a level where I wasn't aware of standards for quoting. I read research from the internet which, I have to admit, was very limited, but if I haven't acknowledged someone's effort I apologise.

PTSD – HIV/AIDS Presentation, 2004

I feel a need to explain before I start this talk properly to tell you that I was diagnosed HIV positive on the 28th of November 1993. I was given approximately 6 months to 2 years to live, at which I laughed. My reply to the Doctor was "So you are telling me that I'm not going to get hit by a bus in the next 6 months." I didn't go back to him.

I felt as if I'd been in a war. I had been wounded and I carried my battle scars with pride. At this stage I had buried over 50 of my friends in six years and as my story unfolds was to bury over 30 more.

My parents and I became involved in a halfway house that was set up for people living with HIV/AIDS (PLWHA) who also were drug and alcohol dependant. We met many friends through St Francis House in Melbourne who, as time went by started to pass away. A fantastic network was set up through this house and I was to learn a lot about how compassionate and hateful people can be to each other.

The predominant arrival of HIV/AIDS in the mid 1980's was such a thing that modern society had never seen. A meaningless slaughter of predominantly young men who were in the prime of their lives.

Not since the Spanish Flu of 1919, which wiped out nearly ¼ of the world's population had science and medicine been totally stupefied and useless in its onslaught and carnage. The comparison has been made to a war because it was all the young men but the contemporary media coined the phrase' Gay Plague". It just so happened that a majority of the people succumbing to the disease were homosexually active men. The connection to IV drug users was to come a bit later. It is interesting to note that because it seemed to be affecting gay men on a majority, heterosexual IV drug users, haemophiliacs and women were not considered to have the same condition that these men had so therefore misdiagnosis was common and access to treatment denied and services were denied because they couldn't have had the same thing.

Just as in the case of war veterans it is only in recent times when PTSD and HIV/AIDS are beginning to be connected. This is called a comorbidity which is medical conditions existing simultaneously and usually independent of each other.

It could be said that anyone who was affected by or involved with the gay community during the epidemic of AIDS from the mid 1980's to the mid 1990's could easily suffer from PTSD. Thousands of lives in Australia were lost during this time. Social bigotry was rife. Family and friends who wanted to be involved became fulltime carers of loved ones who died in the vilest of ways. And there were the workers in the field who suffered with clients over and over falling to their graves.

Persons with HIV/AIDS experienced a range of social, emotional and psychiatric problems. When diagnosed, patients had to deal with having a contagious and progressively debilitating illness as well as rejection and ostracism by society in general. Being diagnosed as HIV positive matches other medical conditions because of its chronic course and other stressful experiences that can occur as part of the disease treatment or context. Also many experienced physical harm by a person close to them as a direct result of their diagnosis. Research has suggested that physicians have even less knowledge of anxiety disorders than of depression. It is PTSD that arises in response to experiencing traumatic life events.

HIV/AIDS related illness, cancer and other chronic life threatening illnesses are characterised by often drawn out periods of treatment and disease free survival. Knowledge about disease reoccurrence can produce greater PTSD symptoms compared to the initial diagnosis if the degree of life threat is considered more intense.

If the focus of threat of life is not based on a past event for medical patients but is based on the future the intrusions and re-experiencing symptoms that occur as part of PTSD syndromes may be of a different type than those experienced by individuals exposed to traditional traumas. The re-experiencing symptom cluster of PTSD is based on past trauma exposure rather than future orientated events.

Symptoms of this cluster could be, for example:

- Flashbacks to the event
- Feeling it's all happening again
- Recurrent distressing dreams
- Cues in your environment that trigger emotional outbursts
- Cues may come from thinking about the future – will I see my family grow?
- Will the disease progress to such a point of so much pain I'll want to die?

Trauma can affect both psychological and physical functioning of the immune system and increase susceptibility to infections. Psychological effects can manifest in risk taking behaviour. People with HIV/AIDS maybe affected past trauma to the point it manifests in problems with disease management such as disrupted or negative interactions with medical personnel and or medication non adherence. Psychological symptoms that commonly occur following a traumatic event will remit spontaneously over time for most people, some researchers believe PTSD as a disorder of recovery.

The likelihood of a patient developing PTSD varies according to the vulnerability of the affected person and the severity of the stressor. A study done in 1996 of 1489 patients with HIV infection 10.4% were diagnosed with

START WITH YOUR OWN ONION

PTSD. Onset of a severe life threatening illness such as HIV/AIDS can sometimes in itself lead to PTSD more often a history of physical and psychological trauma and diagnosis of PTSD co-occurs with an individual's HIV status.

Patients with PTSD may have dissociative symptoms which may be mistaken for HIV related dementia or other neuropsychiatric disorders.

To round up all the technical gibberish I leave you with a personal statement of two dear friends.

Phillip has been HIV positive for over 20 years, and has seen over 100 friends die. At the moment, he is having bad sciatica pain, as well as having dementia related issues, chronic insomnia, abscesses on his back and lips, whose CD_4 count has recently dropped for no apparent reason, as well as his muscle density test - is not panicking but feels shithouse. Phillip is a full-time carer for his beautiful partner Michael who deals with HIV related dementia, epilepsy, encephalitis (brain infection), toxoplasmosis, meningococcal meningitis, deep vein thrombosis and pulmonary embolisms (blood clots in the lungs). Michael has also lost many friends but due to the dementia can't remember though. These two men are happy, in love and are still laughing.

* * *

I have carried around a polystyrene box that I covered in decoupage in 1997. The box was used for a particular nasty drug called Ritonivir, which had to be refrigerated wherever you went. I was put on four drugs in those days. The four together were called "combination therapy". The only previous drug was called AZT and I believe it killed more people than it helped; it was an old cancer drug from the 1950's that didn't work on cancer, so they pulled it out hoping it would work on HIV/AIDS. My box is covered in the colours of fire with pictures of semi-naked firemen taken from calendars, HIV medicine references, a statistic graph showing the dramatic decline of AIDS deaths in San Francisco from 1990 to 1997, an article on the benefits of cannabis on people with HIV, body mind and spirit references to healing, a Sci-Fi character who was part human part technology, and a picture of a friend that I put on the box because he had recently died.

He represented to me everyone who had gone before me. He was a lovely guy full of life when I met him and he had a lovely partner. It wasn't long before his health started to deteriorate and he had to walk with a walking stick. I remember seeing him in Lismore around the ACON offices and functions that we had. They were important events, the lunches. It was very much in amongst The War Years and these groups of people, mainly gay men of very different socio economic backgrounds, possibly never would have mixed except for the virus entering our lives. They were important gatherings to exchange information about treatments, mutual support and check what was happening to everyone at the time.

I recently got the box out of the cupboard and have been, well, not torturing myself, but letting the memories come to me in hope of writing something of value. There's a lot that this box has triggered in my memory and the most significant at the moment is the fact I can't remember the name of the man on the box who was my friend, who passed away nearly twenty years ago. He has almost become a symbol of a somewhat blocked period of my life that I have the most difficulty unravelling. There are so many names I can't remember.

I can see their faces, I can remember horrible growths across beautiful faces, I can remember flesh eating bacteria, Kaposi's Sarcoma across bodies and faces, I can even remember madness, but it's their names that have gone. In a way I feel like I have betrayed them by forgetting, but I also feel there must be a self-preservation factor involved. Two, three or more funerals a week for months or years is somewhat overwhelming, and I got overwhelmed for a while. I sometimes still get a bit overwhelmed.

The combination therapy that I started treatment on was *Ritonivir, Saquinivir, Lamivudine* and S*tavudine* – the worst combination I've had. Five years after diagnosis. It was early days, I hadn't seen proof that people were actually living from this therapy. Some people didn't get side effects. Lucky bastards!

Leaving the pharmacist to go home, the drugs needed to be in the box with an ice block in it. If you wanted to go out anywhere, you needed to prepare the box. If you were to be away at meal time, the medication went with you. Medications had to be taken with food (especially grapefruit) and some needed to be taken an hour after food. One of the first side effects that this combination hit me with was a strange, vile, metallic taste that overwhelmed my mouth. My mouth tingled offensively with this taste. My senses of touch and sight were deadened. Nausea was the new norm, as well as chronic diarrhea. Losing senses like taste and smell, which are vital in cooking, meant I had to stop the job that I had spent most of my teens and adult life doing. I lost the ability to trust my own senses.

I started the medication the first week of January, 1997. The first function I braved away from home was on the 17th;

my dear friend Robyn's 50th birthday. I felt very nauseous that evening and realised I had better not stay too long because the frequency I was having to use the toilet was a bit too obvious. No amount of air freshener was killing the smell of what was coming out of me.

I developed a fear of being far away from the toilet. At Gretel Farm it was not so much of an issue. If I lost myself in the middle of the paddock (the loo was in the main house) it was relatively less embarrassing in front of the horse than if I was in town and a sudden bout of the runs happened. It was very humiliating.

This medication regime demanded a huge price from me: the ability to eat normally and have normal body functions, for many years to come. That, I shall say, "did my head in". It plays upon the reality of quality versus quantity of life. If this was going to be my life, the former was losing huge ground, and the latter became less important every day.

Now, nearly 20 years since the box was used, it's a keepsake of different times. A little sign post of where I have been and where I am now. I do enjoy the "now" and I am proud of where I've come from.

* * *

Best Chocolate Fudge (Thanks Toby)

This is a no brainer without the hassle and expertise of real fudge making and has a great result.

Approximately 500gm of chocolate – I prefer the dark chocolate
1 tin of condensed milk

Toasted nuts or whatever bits you want in it.

- Put ingredients into a crock pot set on medium for an hour
- Stir well
- If it has separated, then you can add a tablespoon of cream and stir well (repeat if necessary to bring it back together)
- Add nuts or bits stir
- Scoop out onto a dish lined with greaseproof paper level it out and let it set
- Cut up and eat.

* * *

Lemon Cordial

Any citrus can be used instead of lemons. Blood oranges have such a short life at the market they make a great flavour and colour cordial. 5 lemons are really the lowest quantity you can use for a satisfactory drink. It is tempting to double the mixture, but I have found that you lose something in the end result. Beware of the citric acid as this can have a bitter taste to the end product. It is needed as a preservative, but you can get away with using ¼ less. If you are making the cordial for a special event, and it will be used in a few days, you can omit the citric acid altogether as long as it's kept in the fridge. I stress: a few days' means about a week. If something has gone wrong, you should know by observation – don't drink if it's bubbling!

At least 5 lemons (decent size lemons or the equivalent in size to other fruits)

1 ½ oz citric acid
2 pints of almost boiling water
2lb sugar

- Peel zest from lemons with a vegetable peeler
- Cut away pith (the white stuff) from the flesh
- Slice lemons
- Add sugar, citric acid and water
- Let stand for 24 hours
- Check to make sure all sugar is dissolved
- Strain and bottle up
- I tend to keep in fridge
- As a little treat, you can add 2/3 of a bottle of vodka to 1/3 cordial and let stand for a week or so.

* * *

Marshmallows

- Dissolve a tablespoon of gelatine in ½ cup of hot water in a saucepan
- Then add 1 cup sugar, bring to boil make sure all is dissolved
- When coolish (about body temperature), pour into the mix master and beat on high till fluffy
- Scoop out onto a tray dusted with icing sugar
- Dust the top with icing sugar and, moving quickly, pat down till flat and desired thickness. It will set shortly
- Once set, it can be cut and dusted with more icing sugar

- Store in a tight container. As long as it is air tight it should keep for a long time

* * *

Pear Honey or Sauce
4 pounds (or two kilos) of pears
Water as needed
3 tablespoons of lemon juice
Grated zest
6 cups of sugar

- Peel and grate pears and put this in acidulated (addition of some lemon juice) water
- Combine 6 cups of water, sugar and pears together
- Add zest and water
- Cook for about an hour till a teaspoon dropped on a cold plate doesn't run over the plate. It should more or less sit where it's been placed
- As long as it's in a sealed container, this can keep for a few years and the longer it is the more gorgeous it seems to be
- Ok, it's not honey as we know honey to be; it's more like a sort of jam, but it isn't as thick as a jam can be. It is delicious! It can be used like apple sauce as an accompaniment to roast pork, cold meats or be used in desserts.

* * *

Date Chutney
1 kg dates

750gm sugar
8 tablespoon garlic
350ml vinegar
½ teaspoon cloves
½ teaspoon cinnamon
250gm sultanas
4 teaspoons salt
4 teaspoons ginger
4 teaspoons mustard

- Make sure all the pips are removed from the dates
- Excluding the sultanas and salt, put everything else into a pot and cook on medium heat. Beware that it can catch and burn
- It needs to be cooked till it's thick and chutney-like
- Add the sultanas and salt when you take it off the heat
- This should make about 4 decent sized jars
- A great present and great with curries.

* * *

Mango Chutney

6 large mangoes (if you have to, 1 tin is equal to 1 large mango)
2 large onions, finely chopped
500gm of brown sugar (can use white sugar)
1 ½ cups vinegar (apple cider, plain white, white balsamic, or a mix of pale vinegars can be used depending on what you want as the end result. If

dark vinegar is used you'll end up with very dark chutney, but that's not such a bad thing)
1 tablespoon of seeded mustard (more according to taste)
2 tablespoons of chopped herbs
1kg tomatoes, preferably skinned and deseeded

- Sauté onions till clear
- Add mangoes that have been peeled and roughly chopped
- Then add tomatoes and cook till mixture gets sloppy
- Follow with the sugar and vinegar; now cook till it's thick
- At the very end, before taking off the heat, add the herbs.

* * *

Mum's Chocolate Crunch
4 cups of SR Flour
4 cups of cornflakes
4 cups of coconut
2 cups of brown sugar
½ lb of butter
4 heaped tablespoons of cocoa

- Combine all dry ingredients in a bowl
- Melt the butter and stir through the dry ingredients
- Mix well
- In a lined baking dish, press the mixture onto the tray about 3cm in thickness

- Bake at 150C (300F) for 10-15 minutes
- When baked, let cool before icing
- Coat with chocolate icing, a ganache, and sprinkle the icing with toasted coconut
- Once icing is set, cut into squares.

***

Mum's Raspberry Shortcake

½ cup butter
½ cup sugar
1 egg
2 cups SR flour
2-3 tablespoons of jam (you don't have to use raspberry)

- Combine ingredients together
- Press into a baking tray about 2-3cm thickness
- Spread jam onto dough
- Then combine 1 cup coconut, ¾ cup of sugar, 1 egg
- Put on top of jam
- Bake in a moderate oven till golden brown
- Slice into squares when cool.

***

Mum's Apple Batter Cake

START WITH YOUR OWN ONION

- Melt together 60gm butter and ¾ cup milk
- When cool, add 1 egg
- 1 cup sugar
- Beat well
- Add 1¼ to 1½ cups SR flour
- Make to batter consistency
- Pour the batter onto a greased tray or one that has been lined with baking paper
- Peel and slice two apples and spread them on top of the batter
- Sprinkle with cinnamon sugar
- Bake in a moderate oven till brown
- Pears or any fresh or preserved fruit can be used including berries or nuts of any variety
- Generally, it should be served within a few hours with lashings of cream.

* * *

Engadine

Pate Sable (from chapter two)

- Line a flan tin with an even coating of the dough then put into freezer
- When it's frozen, put into a moderate oven and bake till light brown
- When cool, coat with 100gm melted chocolate
- Caramelise:
- 840gm sugar
- 2/3 cup water
- 1 teaspoon of lemon juice
- 1 teaspoon of spirit, vodka, brandy etc.
- When cool, add:

- 2 cups cream
- 2 eggs and 2 yolks
- ½ cup soft butter
- Spread 3 cups of walnuts onto flan and pour on caramel
- Bake in a slow oven on 130C for ¾ to 1 hour
- It should be set and not show any signs of still being liquid
- When cool, coat with a ganache (melted chocolate and cream – 100gm chocolate to at least 2 tablespoons of cream) and let set
- This will keep for a long time, it's rich and delicious.

* * *

Strawberry Flummery

1 punnet strawberries, hulled and rough chopped
1 punnet strawberries, pureed
600ml cream
¾ cup caster sugar
6 egg whites

- Whip cream, add ½ of the sugar
- Add most of the puree
- Whip whites and add rest of sugar
- Whip till solid peaks
- When firm, fold ½ egg whites through strawberry cream till combined, then add the rest and fold through
- Fold through chopped strawberries and top with the rest of the puree
- Serve relatively quickly.

You can substitute any berries for the strawberries, or make a mix of berries, peaches or any stone fruit. Depending on your taste, it might help to add a few teaspoons of lemon juice or a good blast of booze to the puree just to liven the taste. Crushed biscuits or meringue and of course chocolate in all forms can be folded through and a cap full of liqueur to set it off just before serving!

SEVEN

DON'T LIE AT FUNERALS

At Queenscliff Hotel I had the pleasure of meeting some amazing people. For me, when people hang around in your life or come back after a time it makes life so complete. There was a waitress at Queenscliff that loved chocolate and, being in the cold larder in charge of desserts, she appreciated my goods!

Bronwyn is articulate, softly spoken, incredibly diplomatic in her behaviour, very well educated, pretty unflappable, and most importantly: as a waitress, her dockets were always clearly written, and she remembered where food was meant to go! There's nothing worse than a soufflé going to the wrong table!

Many times, even the most controlled person can "have a moment" during a stressful service. I'm sure Bronwyn believes that she did "lose it" at some stage – but I never saw it. The type of clientele that the hotel attracted was usually a demanding, privileged group in the socioeconomic sphere. I remember looking forward to the weekend crew coming down to the hotel. Bronwyn was part of a mixed bag of local and international waiters from some of the finer restaurants

START WITH YOUR OWN ONION

in Melbourne and beyond. The staff, both floor and kitchen, were very cosmopolitan.

One of the teams I worked with included Michael (the crayfish in brioche man), he was Irish, the second chef (Annesley) was from Sri Lanka. We had Ivana from Italy, who came and made our pasta twice a week and Tim, the uncoordinated and often frowned upon apprentice, and of course Eileen in the scullery.

On the eve of Tim getting dismissed, Michael put him into the position of calling orders. This was the centre of a busy kitchen and during the service, suddenly he seemed to get "it". The service was a joy to be part of and at a reunion over a decade later, was remembered very affectionately. He owned his power and everything went without a flaw. It was like watching the boy become a man over a period of several hours. Needless to say, Tim didn't get sacked and went on to become a fine chef.

There were Japanese, French and quite a few other nationalities in the kitchen. I was introduced to many different types of food, and expectations (even on myself) were very high. As bosses go, Patricia was possibly the most knowledgeable on food and service that I have ever met coming from a family hospitality dynasty.

Huge bowls of flowers greeted guests as they walked in the foyer. Lots of stained glass was restored (most of which had to be bought back from locals during the reconstruction phase), bright orange linoleum from the 70's had been ripped up to discover beautiful Italian tiles underneath, and the paint work was based on original designs.

Around this time, the late 1980's, Bronwyn and I went to warehouse parties, we went clubbing, had dinner parties – she always made you feel like you were the most important person with her optimistic manner. It's her genuine personality that I really warmed to. As I said, Bronwyn loved chocolate, and the expressions on her face whenever I gave her a sample of something I had created were worth taking photos of. Unfortunately, I never did. These were the days before "selfies".

When I moved to NSW and opened the restaurant, communication with just about all my friends in Victoria became less frequent. *SUGI'S* lasted for about 18 months, then I took a job at a restaurant in Byron in 1993 – a funny place called *"The Rocks"* and, in a way, it might as well have been on the rocks. The owners of the motel and restaurant were, as a lot of owners are, not particularly informed about things – especially running restaurants.

Not surprisingly, I met some great people there. One in particular has been a dear friend to this day; I call her Princess Robyn. She was a house keeper and also cared for her mother, Thora. My job there went well for a while but inevitably turned sour. I was given the sack on a Friday then the following Monday, November 28th 1993, I was diagnosed with HIV – so I'm glad that I didn't have to deal with work.

Looking back on so many different periods in my life, I have often been surrounded by strong and powerful women – all of whom I have affectionately called my "Earth Mother Goddesses". Robyn was indeed a very important member of that group.

* * *

A couple of months after my diagnosis, dealing with the thought of my mortality, I decided it was time I told Mum and Dad. As far as I was concerned, they deserved to know if there was a chance I wasn't going to make it. They had been so amazing doing volunteer work for HIV positive people from about 1986 till the early 90's. These were the days before medication and all of the people they cared for were basically dying people. A lot of them had been discarded by biological family and had nowhere else to go. Many had drug and alcohol issues, and my very brave parents became surrogate parents for these (mainly) men who were dying.

My very-Catholic parents. I say that because Catholics get a bit of a hard time – and fair enough, a lot of awful things have happened; but the nuns who helped set up and assist in the ongoing maintenance of St Francis House (and the volunteers, including my parents) were, and are, amazing.

***

I had seen so much anger and bullshit around parents' reactions to the triple whammy. One: your son is dying, two: your son is gay, and three: your son is dying of AIDS.

So much anger came bursting out of people. In a way, it's hard to blame some parents for reacting (to a point) the way they did, for it was hard for anybody to deal with. On the other hand, if you hadn't been a bigoted dick in the first place and kicked your son out of home, or disowned your son, or just not bothered to talk to your son for years then, in a way, you reap what you sow.

One develops theories when one does things regularly – and funerals, I was doing regularly. I often thought the final act of betrayal by parents was not even bothering to attend their child's funeral. Then I encountered a dear friend's death, and as his body was being lowered into its resting place, his father walked up to the edge of the grave and spat on the coffin. There was nearly a riot and I can't understand why he bothered to attend in the first place. To me, this cuts through the very fabric of what is a decent human being.

Petty, morally bankrupt people. These parents and relatives of the deceased went about contesting wills. There were no laws in place for significant others. Biological families who hadn't spoken to their sons in years forced away the very people that had cared and nurtured their offspring. These relatives came in and, through long legal action, basically made the loved partner homeless.

Grieving spouses, who had also been carers, were often not well themselves, had put in half of the assets, had lost their lover and, because of greedy lowlifes, had also lost their homes.

For this reason I support the idea of same-sex marriage; that if two people make a legally binding contract, the contract should be honoured. It's as simple as that! I don't believe it needs to have the same guilt-ridden dramas that heterosexuals often base a relationship on.

I've felt so much contempt for so-called "normal heterosexual" human beings who are called parents (who are often that in name only). The reality is, they didn't parent respectfully at all. Their sons were not cold in the ground when the legal action began. So much hate that ripped apart grieving partner's lives. The lover who had just lost his love – and was forced to lose his home.

I remember attending a morning funeral and, afterwards, a small wake held back at the home of the deceased and his partner. The parents attended the funeral and were invited back to the house. They arrived with a removalist truck and immediately started badgering the partner; demanding attention as to their sons' possessions. As soon as the truck was full and the parents were satisfied they had their booty, they and the truck left. There was no offer to help with finances for burying their son.

During this time I resolved that not everyone has the right to breed. Gay or straight, not everyone has a right, because with rights comes responsibilities.

These so-called parents left their responsibilities at the door barged into the house like savages demanding loot.

March, 1994

My dear friend Elizabeth, who I'd met at BayFM, and her then partner Phillip, took me to the train station at Byron. The station is connected rather conveniently to one of the Byron pubs – so it was a great place to bid farewell. I took the train to Sydney where I had a twelve hour wait at Central Station before catching the train to Melbourne.

By chance, I bumped into Bronwyn, who happened to be on the same train going to Melbourne. It was such an incredible moment. I tried to get seats changed, but unfortunately that couldn't happen. To this day, I can remember seeing her sitting about ten rows in front of me and I feeling a great sense of security.

Naturally, I was feeling every emotion under the sun. I was preparing to tell Mum and Dad that I may die – but I was determined to live. My emotions were scattered and I was on the point of bursting into tears for the whole journey.

Bronwyn was going to Germany to study, and was uncertain where she would be. I eventually was to return to Byron – homeless. My things were in storage. We had little chats on the train, but I couldn't focus. I wanted to talk and organise things but I just couldn't get my head around the details. My job at hand was just too big without trying to add anything else. I told Bronwyn about my diagnosis, but omitted that I had been given a timeframe.

Maybe this was the last time we would see each other, maybe not. Mum and Dad were picking me up at the station. I desperately didn't want to look like an emotional wreck. The train pulled into Spencer St. I hugged Bronwyn goodbye and Mum and Dad hello. I gave little introductions on the platform, but Mum and Dad were anxious to get me home.

As we drove, there were so many things that went through my head that I could have – should have – said if only I had been more focused. The one thing I really wanted to say to Bronwyn was that our chance meeting on that train trip was so incredibly powerful for me. Although I couldn't speak much, I so believed that I had an angel on the train looking after me. It was far too coincidental; far too serendipitous for me, and has had a significant impact on my belief system.

For years I wanted to tell Bronwyn that having a friend, just being there, on that train was so powerful that I believed my gods were looking after me.

2013

I had learnt to Google people's names and see what came up. I'd done internet searches on Bronwyn in the past, but had never found anything. I used Google to find out Mitchell was dead. My posting on Facebook got a huge response that day: *"Is it ok to scream whoopee and have a little dance when you find out an abusive partner who broke bones and many possessions is dead?"*

I thought of old school people and found one or two – then what about Bronwyn? I Googled again, and up popped the same gorgeous face, not looking in any way as though twenty years had gone by.

I grabbed the phone and rang the number. I spoke to a receptionist who said the message would be passed on. It was about a week later, and I had sort of given up a bit of hope, when I received an SMS from Bronwyn saying that she was in the States and would be home soon – and wanted to catch up.

Sitting in a fabulous little restaurant and being able to tell Bronwyn what I had wanted to say for 20 years was a defining moment for me.

'The chance meeting in Sydney, when we had last met was just so important. I knew what I had to do – and to have a friend, just around me, seemed like I was being protected. How do you thank someone for being in the exact right place at the exact right time?'

I felt as if I could have quite easily died there and then; that life would have made all the sense it needed to at that particular moment. It was a full circle moment – a completion of a task that seemed would never eventuate.

Bronwyn asked during our first phone conversation if I still made a certain cake that she loved at Queenscliff. I had to pull the recipe out of the deep dark recesses and after dinner at the restaurant we went back to her place for dessert and more catching up on 20 years.

* * *

Chocolate Whiskey Raisin Cake

225gm almond meal
6 eggs
300gm sugar
400gm dark chocolate

90ml water
225gm butter
50gm SR flour
50gm plain flour
½ cup raisins
½ cup whiskey
A pinch of baking powder

- Soak the raisins in the whiskey and water
- This can be done a day before – a week before depending on how organised you are. Soaked raisins will last in the fridge for months and they are a tasty after dinner snack in their own right
- Melt the chocolate and butter together
- Separate the eggs
- Whip most of the sugar and yolks together
- Add chocolate mixture
- Fold through almond meal and sifted together flours and baking powder
- Whip whites and rest of sugar together to form stiff peaks
- Fold into the mixture in two goes
- Pour into a tin lined with greaseproof paper. This needs to be a solid one piece cake tin, not a ring tin.
- Bake in a bain-marie in a moderate oven for about ¾ hour.

***

I learnt a thing or two about my own arrogant ways which caused a bit of personal family displeasure. I was asked to make a family members wedding cake. The stipulation was no "squidgy bits". Squidgy implied any dried fruit. I was arrogant and not respectful enough to not adhere to the brief. I thought I knew better and made this cake thinking it was going to be okay. Well it sort of wasn't. What can I say; the guests liked it, BUT, that wasn't the brief. I'm truly sorry. Moral of this short story: When people ask for specifics - do what they ask! It's not good to assume anything.

* * *

1990
I made this chocolate cake at a hotel I worked at on the "right side of town" where there were too many owners, most of whom didn't do much work – but they did like to party.

I was the pastry chef and I was asked to make a wedding cake for one of the bosses. I offered several cake options to the part-owner and his wife-to-be and they chose the chocolate whiskey cake. The wedding reception was for about 200 people, and they wanted 200 serves in one cake, which I wasn't fond of. For a big party there's the cake on show and you prepare the rest in the kitchen. A 200-serve cake is just showing off. I didn't enjoy making something so vulgar; they wanted it big, showy and over the top.

They asked for royal icing so it became a big meringue thing with rose petals and ribbons. I spent about two days making the cakes to assemble this monster. I think there was something like six bottles of scotch used.

I had to come into work on my day off to help with the service, and after the main courses were served I was able to go home. We all witnessed a lot of the food come back – but everyone said the food was fabulous.

We observed hardly any of the food was touched – entrées or main courses.

The chef was a bit of a contemptible thing, but he was screaming 'Coke addicts! Fucking idiots!'

I left before dessert because there were enough staff members on.

I came in on the Monday and the cake had been thrown in the bin. I asked what he story was and was told they forgot to serve it, so the chef threw it out. I said: 'If you didn't like it – surely I could have taken it down to a soup kitchen?'

'No. Get to work.'

I have witnessed appalling waste in the hospitality industry. It sickens me. I love the idea that organisations like *Oz Harvest* are able to tap into this disgraceful excess.

I went on to see a few functions of a similar nature. All the "guests" would be doing strange things with rolled up notes on the table at a wedding, and wouldn't touch their food. It was times like this in life when a random idiot with a gun would have been a good thing. I was pretty angry during this time.

1991

When I worked at *Society* the owners were a couple of solicitors who had no idea about running a restaurant and behaved really badly. While I was there, my recipe book mysteriously "disappeared" – the book I had written the most important recipes in. It had a collection of many friends' hand-written recipes, including Nana Young's Fruit

START WITH YOUR OWN ONION

Cake. I was very upset. I ran around the place virtually looking for my left arm!

I'd been in the office causing a bit of commotion and the owner told me if I didn't stop pestering him, he knew people that would put me in cement shoes.

I said: 'You'd kill me over my recipe book? Why don't you just photo copy it?' I looked at the photocopy machine and there it was – being photocopied. I was sacked, but sort of resigned at the same time.

Another time, my book was "misplaced" was at a restaurant owned by a family who I think just had a lot of money. This was an opportunity to work with Roger Fowler again (who I worked with at Queenscliff Hotel). The restaurant was not far from my home. The owners were stalwarts of the 1970's who tried a little to modernise in the 90's.

The rather loud bully second chef was a fan of Queen the band, but he wasn't fond of queens the men. He refused to believe that Freddy Mercury was gay. I laughed so hard about that, he got very upset and the more upset he became the more I laughed.

The matriarch of the family owners said to one of the waitress's (in a heavy European accent): 'Darling, I like your silver ring, but I prefer zee gold.'

That line became a bit of a catch cry. This matriarch made the cakes for the dessert trolley. We called them cakes to her face but behind her back they were called hockey pucks. I've never known harder fruit flans in all my life. I was the pastry cold larder person, and there was a time when she was sick and couldn't do the cakes – so I was given the job. Everyone was surprised when we started selling cakes. When she got better I was in a swing of making a few things and we just added her flans to the trolley. She started getting a bit shitty about some of her cakes not selling – but all mine did.

There was a bit of a conference; she wanted to know why her cakes weren't selling. She involved the waiters and the chef and her family. Everyone said that her cakes were great and she believed them, of course.

After the rather humiliating intervention, I decided to do something naughty. When the family had left, the chef and floor staff were stating the obvious: that her cakes were shithouse.

I said: 'Do you know why her cakes don't sell?' They looked at me and I picked up one her flans, and threw it against the wall. Remarkably, it stayed together and fell onto the floor in two bits. 'That's why!'

Everyone burst out laughing and the daughter with bad skin and flaming curls came into the kitchen, just as I had picked up the tart from the floor.

She had an expression on her face that said she knew she had just missed something. She asked for my recipe book, which I gave her. It was a Saturday night – and on Monday morning when I asked for it back she replied that she did not know what I was talking about. She then threatened me with the police.

I went to the chef and asked him if he remembered me giving her the book. He didn't, but the kitchen hand did. I was glad I wasn't going insane.

It was obvious I was going to be sacked, so I went to the public telephone within earshot of the daughter and called the police. I didn't really, but followed through on a pretend-conversation I was having with them. I was fully intending on going to the police but wanted to get the wind up her.

Only a few minutes later, she handed me the book and

said that she had found it in the restaurant. I only went back for my last pay.

***

Another person I worked for was in the tropics on Hamilton Island. He was the financier of a dear friend Joanne who had started a business, and we had worked there for about a year. Her position became untenable and she left. I was left with a skeleton staff and a resentful, nasty owner. His wife would come into the restaurant to work on the till occasionally with a black eye, where she had "fallen into a door".

I had to go to a dear friend's funeral, Robby Harkness; his death was a shock to everyone. I flew to Byron.

When I got back, the owner was in a filthy mood. He immediately started telling me that I was doing a bad job – or some such thing, and I said to him: 'I will organise whatever is needed. If I could just have an hour before I start work I've just been to a funeral.'

'Well, we all know what he died from, don't we?'

'I beg your pardon?'

'Bloody poofs getting this AIDS – they probably deserve it!'

I walked back to the unit and thought about what he had said and gave him my resignation. He said: 'You can't go now! I can make it very difficult for you!'

'Yeah, as if. And by the way, Robby died of throat cancer.'

He did try to give me a hard time. Inspectors arrived and came into my unit. A palette arrived for me to put my things on and I was escorted off the island. I pretended it was a farewell committee. I was glad to get off. My stereo disappeared in transit as well as a few other items. The days weren't all bad there. I cooked for and waved hello to George Harrison. He was pleased I knew what a vegan was and I cooked a couple of things for him. That was nice.

***

Joanne's Apricot Sherbet
   1 ¼ cups lemon juice
   2 cups sugar
   1 476gm tin of apricots drained and pureed
   1 600ml half milk and half cream

- Combine all ingredients. Make sure it has a good sweet/lemon balance
- Now churn in an ice cream machine or;
- Place in the freezer till semi-frozen, then take out and stir it all through, making sure liquids aren't settling into layers
- Place back in the freezer
- Stir it through over into itself a few times, maybe three times in the first hour or so
- This reduces large icicles forming.

***

Muesli
   500gm sultanas
   500gm dates, dried
   500gm apricots, dried
   500gm figs, dried
   500gm pears, dried
   250gm sunflower seeds
   200gm oat bran

500gm rye flakes
1kg shredded coconut
1kg walnuts, chopped
500gm wheat flakes
1kg rolled oats
250gm pepitas
1 cup brown sugar
2 large kitchen spoons honey

This is a base recipe. A loose guide to however you like your end result. Toasting everything means that you lay it out on a tray at a pretty even level and bake in a moderate oven about 180C till there is some colour. In a health food store I've seen at least six different rolled grains as well as all sorts of things not mentioned in the recipe (LSA, psyllium, rice bran, etc.).

- When doing large volumes I toast individual ingredients just till they all start to brown
- Be careful not to darken them as everything does get a second bake
- I do not toast the dried fruit or the puffed things rice, millet, chia etc. at this stage
- Once all ingredients are toasted and cool they can be tossed together
- The honey, treacle, golden syrup and sugar (or combinations of) are brought together over a heat till the sugar dissolves
- Once this is done, let it cool and pour over the toasted ingredients
- Once it's all rubbed through, the muesli is again

placed on trays and baked again for about 10 minutes
- Let completely cool before packing away
- This can keep in sealed jars for many weeks.

* * *

My Chocolate Pudding

In my handwritten recipe book I've somehow called this "My Pudding". Truthfully, I can't remember its development – it's lost to history, but it's a bit of a winner!

125gm butter
    100gm brown sugar
    2 eggs
    50gm plain flour
    50gm SR flour
    250gm chocolate
    ½ cup whiskey, spirit or orange juice
    125gm double cream

- Cream butter and most of the sugar
- Add yolks
- Melt the cream and chocolate together and add to the butter keep beating
- Sift the flours together and carefully combine in the mix
- Add the liquid
- Whip the whites with the rest of the sugar and fold through the mix
- Bake in a bain-marie (that's the roasting tray with hot water in it)

- Approximately ½ hr to ¾ hour moderate oven
- Serve with lashings of cream and strawberries

Note: to make this a gluten free pudding, use dark chocolate. The ratio to replace flour is 3 cups almond and 2 teaspoons baking powder = 1 cup SR flour.

* * *

Mum's Boiled Chocolate Cake

This is another base recipe that can be played around with. I have substituted spirit or orange juice for the water. I've used honey, brown sugar, treacle or combinations of instead of the plain white sugar. Also for the flour I have substituted 3 cups of nut meal to make it gluten free. I have a preference for a silky textured cake so this can be achieved by following the bain-marie method described above. If you want a cake that is to be layered like a Black Forest, it's best not to cook this way. Simply bake in the oven. This method will give you a more firm texture and solid consistency. If left to stand for a day it will cut with ease and will lap up the boozy sugar syrup you splash on it.

4oz butter
1 ½ cups sugar
1 cup water
2 tablespoon cocoa

- Boil the above ingredients together

- When the mix comes to the boil add ½ teaspoon bi carb
- Allow to fizz
- Let the mix cool
- Whip through the 2 eggs
- Add 1 ½ cups SR flour and beat till smooth
- Approx. 1 hour in 325F oven

The eggs can be separated first add the yolks at the mentioned egg stage and the whipped whites folded through as the last step after the flour. Always fold through whipped whites like this in two stages.

* * *

Shane's Beetroot and Chocolate Cake

250gm butter
250gm sugar
375gm dark chocolate
6 eggs, one at a time
2 large beetroots peeled and grated
250gm SR flour

- Melt chocolate, setting aside 75gm that is to be used for the ganache (the chocolate icing)
- Whip butter sugar till light in colour add melted chocolate
- Fold through eggs and flour and beetroot
- Bake moderate oven for about an hour till firm in the centre to touch.

* * *

Fudge Chocolate Brownies
125gm unsalted butter
90gm dark chocolate
90gm milk chocolate
½ cup brown sugar
2 tablespoons honey
2 eggs
1 cup plain flour
2/3 cup unsalted macadamias or nuts

- This will make a sufficient amount for a 20cm x 20cm tin
- Line the baking tin with greaseproof paper
- Melt chocolates and butter together
- Dissolve sugar and honey together over low heat and let cool
- Stir in sugar and honey
- Stir in eggs
- Then flour and nuts
- Bake in moderate oven in bain-marie
- Cool in pan and cut when cold.

* * *

Dining Room Chocolate Cake
½ lb butter
225gm chocolate
2 tablespoons milk
¼ lb almond meal
6 tablespoons sugar
6 eggs, separated

- Do not use a ring tin, this needs to be a solid one piece tin. Line the cake tin with baking paper and prepare a bain-marie (roasting tray, half filled with water, in the oven)
- Melt the chocolate and butter together
- Then add the milk (making sure the milk is not too cold because you will solidify the chocolate)
- Whisk the yolks and 5 tablespoons of sugar together till light in colour and well combined
- Add the chocolate mix to the yolks
- Fold the almond meal through
- Whisk the whites till light and fluffy adding the last tablespoon of sugar and keep whipping till sugar is dissolved and meringue is firm
- Fold ¼ of the whites through the chocolate, mix till well combined then fold through the rest of the whites
- Pour mix into the cake tin put into bain-marie and bake in a moderate (160-180C) oven for 35 to 45 minutes
- Cake is baked when firm to touch in the centre
- Let it cool in the tin before turning out onto a plate.

***

Chocolate Marquis

220gm dark chocolate
10 yolks
325gm castor sugar
450gm butter, room temperature
250gm cocoa
750ml cream

75gm icing sugar

- Prepare a loaf tin lined with baking paper or silicon mould
- Melt chocolate
- Whip egg yolks and sugar well
- Add to chocolate
- Beat the soft butter and cocoa together then add the melted chocolate mix
- Whip the cream till soft and fluffy but stands up. Be careful not to over whip it doesn't need to be stiff
- Once whipped, fold through the chocolate
- This will start to set quickly so beware! It is about making sure the chocolate is not too cool and the cream not too whipped
- Fold the two together. The cream will go in two batches: 1/3 and then 2/3
- Into a loaf tin lined with baking paper, press the chocolate mixture and let set in the fridge. This will last for at least a week in a fridge
- For a different look, you can line the loaf tin with cake or biscuits
- This is a really rich dessert and can be served with fruit dressed in booze or some crème fraiche, good plain yoghurt or anything with a strong flavour.

* * *

Chocolate and Macadamia Torte

3 tablespoons of cocoa
¾ cups sugar

2 cups of macadamias, toasted
½ cup of sour cream
350gm chocolate
2 teaspoons vanilla
8 eggs
250gm butter

- Line a 25cm flan tin with pate sable (from Chapter 2) as the base for the torte (it's the 150gm icing sugar, 350gm butter and 500gm flour)
- Mark the pastry with the prongs of a fork, this is to prevent air bubbles forming in the base
- Put it in the freezer to freeze solid
- Straight from there into an moderate oven 180C till it's light golden.

Freezer to oven is done so you don't have to worry about blind baking which is really boring. You cover the pastry with paper then rice or beans these keep the pastry from bubbling up. So does the freezing so I prefer this method.

- Once this is baked and let cool start with the filling
- Melt the butter and sugar together then add the chocolate. This can be done over a double boiler or I prefer on a low setting in the microwave
- Combine the sour cream and yolks with the vanilla then fold through the chocolate
- Beat the whites till stiff
- Fold half the whipped whites into the chocolate

then add the rest. Just before it's all combined add the macadamias
- This can stand alone without the pastry base
- It can be put into little serving bowls and served with Tuiles or brandy snaps or sweet biscuits
- It can be rolled up in foil lined with baking paper to make a sausage shape and once set it can be unwrapped and sliced
- The marquise and this torte are really rich, a special treat even. Just beware you can overdose on it.

* * *

Mississippi Mud Cake

This can be put together several ways and the outcome is dependent on what you want. If you want an end result that is good to be layered with cream and fruit then its best to follow the first three points in the method. Follow that with the rest of the ingredients and bake in a ring cake tin lined with baking paper for about an hour till firm in the centre. If you want a rich moist light cake then follow the bain-marie method.

250gm butter
150gm chocolate cake
2 cups of sugar
1 cup hot water
1/3 cup whiskey or orange juice
1 tablespoon instant coffee (I tend to use a cup of strong brewed coffee instead of instant and hot water)

¼ cup cocoa

- Melt all ingredients together
- Then add:
- 2 eggs
- 1 cup Self raising flour
- ¾ cup of plain flour
- Dissolve or brew coffee and hot water
- Melt the chocolate and butter together
- Add the whiskey or orange juice
- Add most of the sugar set aside a tablespoon for the whites
- Add the yolks to the chocolate and the flours and any other little bits you'd like to put in (toasted flaked almonds are good)
- Whip whites and add the rest of the sugar
- Fold through the batter and bake in a bain-marie moderate oven. Possibly an hour to an hour ¼
- Let it cool in the tin before placing on a baking rack.

* * *

1994

After a few days at Mum and Dad's, I spent the next few days visiting the rest of the family telling them my news. All received it as I hoped: with love, hugs and a few tears. There is something sort of anti-climactic about knowing you have done the hardest thing you will ever have to do in your life. That being said, it is somewhat comforting to be able to get that out of the way.

My journey to Melbourne was clear in intention; I

needed to tell Mum and Dad that I was diagnosed. The time frame was ticking, it had been four months since my diagnosis with six months to no more than two years as my timeframe, and as brave or stupid as I felt, I was determined to live longer than the time I had been given. I did not want to be the ravaged corpse, in a hospital bed like those dear men my parents had encountered during their time at St Francis House.

I hadn't seen Mum and Dad in over a year. I had so much respect and love for what they had done and were doing as volunteers in the HIV sector. I still tell of their deeds to this day, and hear nothing but praise for the sort of people they are.

I was not going to tell anyone timeframes handed out by the doctor. I believe what HIV meant for me was a chemical reaction that happens in a test tube. I wouldn't let "facts" define my existence and predetermine my future. Blood results were not up to date or as refined as they are today. The sample of blood taken was a representation of what happened two or three weeks prior to receiving the news. Such vagaries had to be given some conscious thought, but I refused to let them over take my life. For example, at one stage I had 200 t-cells, then I got PCP (pneumonia) and my t-cells jumped to a massive 800. Never before had I had them so high! As sick as I was, it made me laugh that well.

I'm going to get through this because the blood results implied that I was in good or excellent health.

About two months later I got over the PCP and had more bloods taken, the results were a slightly crushing 200 again. My doctor explained that the possible reason was that during my sickness my body had pulled out "all the stops" to combat the illness. 200 being a "normal" level of health (which isn't all that good) and 800 was in reserve. I came to the conclusion after a while that what will be will be; what was happening in the moment was the priority focus. I fought and – in a way – won a small battle with this virus.

For me this moment was vital. I needed them – my Mum and Dad – like I had never needed anyone before in my life. They didn't disappoint in any way. They had always been my shoulder to cry on throughout all the deaths that had been going on (and continued to go on), and it seemed on some spiritual cosmic level they had done all this volunteer work to help them get their head around what I was going to tell them.

I can choose to believe that life is just a random chance event based on the fact that two molecules crashed into each other 15 billion years ago and that is it – or I can choose to believe I am blessed, loved and that this game we play called life has a meaning far greater than the equation of what makes the sum of us.

***

Chicken and Vegetable Soup

- Chicken stock from *Clements Hainan Chicken* (possibly minus the star anise)
- Sauté some onions and garlic in a pot
- Add diced carrot potato celery capsicum, adding one vegetable at a time, cooking well
- Add broth to how ever many you are cooking for so you have enough for a bowl full for each person
- Cook slowly if you have the time, but it can be rapid boiled if making a quick meal. The idea is

not to boil your spuds till they are mushy. I like a still-together potato in soup
- Taste and season
- There are so many things that can tart up this simple stock soup:
- By adding a good dessertspoon of aioli, pesto, any sort of medium chopped antipasto vegetable, a few capers, small cubes or grated cheese, crusty croutons, a small handful of crispy fried onions, chopped herbs of any sort, lots of basil, spring onion, parsley, coriander (use less of the stronger herbs rosemary sage or thyme)
- There are some wonderful finishing salts like truffle salt, black lava salt, amazing herb-infused salts are around. Put some coriander or fennel seeds or dried mint into a pestle and grind them with some rock salt
- I enjoy roughly chopping some iceberg lettuce, rocket, radicchio or maybe some Chinese greens, putting a small handful into the bowl, and pouring a ladle of soup over the fresh greens.

* * *

I wanted to have a meal with Mum and Dad, something special. I needed to share with them. Mum decided she wanted to invite a friend who was a priest, Fr. Peter Wood. I wasn't sure how I felt about Mum inviting him. He was working within the HIV Catholic response. He was the priest referred to in Timothy Conigrave's *"Holding the Man"*. A book I have a strong affinity with; going to a similar school in suburban Melbourne, probably knowing people that could have known him. We possibly went to the same clubs as young gay men. We would have known similar people working in the sector and this priest.

***

Risotto

- Cook as much risotto rice as needed. For this dish I thought a seafood number would be good. It's not necessary to use all shellfish stock to cook the rice in, so you can cook the rice in mostly water.
- Cook the arborio rice as directed. For 4-6 meals use 2 or 3 cups of prawn stock and rest water. If you use anymore for that amount of rice the flavour can be a bit strong.
- In a separate pot sauté onions and garlic in a pan and quickly add prawns, cubes of fish and whatever fresh seafood you want to add.
- A good handful of dill can be added when seafood is cooked. A glass of wine or some of the stock to boil all the yummy bits off the pan and then stir that through the rice.
- There is a golden rule for purists: not to serve parmesan with seafood. All good rules can be broken if that's your fancy
- A few chopped capers, roast capsicum, semi-dried tomatoes and herbs can be sprinkled on top
- Bocconcini or a soft cheese chopped or broken apart like even knobs of ricotta can be great.

* * *

We had the meal in the dining room, which was a room that was used only for special occasions. I grilled this priest, this Father Wood (call me Peter), on many contentious topics that the church had opinions on. It got to the point where, after the entrée, Dad came to the kitchen where I was preparing main course and told me to pull my horns in and stop attacking the man. Maybe Peter felt attacked, I'm not sure. I just didn't want to disclose in front of this man and have a whole diatribe of so-called religious bull come out of his mouth. I needed to be confident in him being able to deal, and he seemed to pass the test.

* * *

Orange and Cardamom Jelly

In warmer weather a good jelly can be made with a clear jelly powder (agar for the vegetarians) or leaf gelatine and flavoured with any juice, fruit, booze, spice or herb imaginable. Maybe an orange jelly made with juice with a sprinkle of cardamom powder and some orange liqueur, topped with a pipe of chocolate mousse, or maybe with a sprinkle of crumbled meringue on top with fresh raspberries.

* * *

During dessert I decided it was now or never. I said that I had been to the doctors and had been given some results. The results were that I had tested positive for HIV.

The "bomb" was dropped and I sat in my seat. I was looking at Mum who was sitting on my left and I saw her face contort and crush. She ran out of the room with a scream, one which I will never forget. It was as if she ran to escape a blast; a blast from a bomb that I was responsible for dropping. Dad, who was to my right, got up and put his hand on my shoulder kept repeating *'Oh Greg, Oh Greg, Oh Greg.'*

Peter, who I was opposite to on the table, looked at me and said: 'I understand what the questions were about. You are a very brave man.'

I'm pretty sure no one had ever called me brave before. I didn't feel whatever brave was supposed to feel like. He went to Mum and they came back a minute or two later and Mum incredibly emotional grabbed me and cried. Unbeknownst to me till many years later, she had to take a month off work after this, dealing with the news.

After a period of time, I can't be certain how long, we all sat and the questions arose about diagnosis and health. I believe I gave as positive attitude as I could. I explained that I had told the rest of the family and that they were all supportive and loving. I also expressed my concern that this news clashed with the fabulous news of my sister Majella's engagement. This was something that really upset me; I felt like the ultimate "grandstander" raining on her parade.

It had to be done and in a way I was relieved that I had done it. Many people have chosen not to tell their parents, and I respect that decision. It just wouldn't have been right for me considering what they had done.

So, very like my coming out at 17 years old, ten years prior, I had to come out again as HIV positive. This coming out had a whole new meaning to the phrase. With the support of Mum, Dad, the rest of my family and my cherished friends I am here today looking better at 50 than I ever did in my 30's. I know that there has been and always will be angels watching over me. Not in a creepy way whilst in intimate moments, but in a way that protects and guides me.

Why I am still here after so many died? Why have I escaped and lived to tell the tale? I can't say because I don't know. All I know is HIV was the greatest cosmic kick in the arse. It gave me the simple question a fundamental question: *do I want to live or die?* Both options equally valid. Whichever one I chose, I had to do it well. By well I mean I had to deal with my insecurities, my fundamental self-doubts, my ability to self-sabotage. I had to dig up as many negative emotions as I could, process, acknowledge and then let go of them.

Counselling has been an essential tool in assisting in clarifying these life issues. Guilt about creating so much pain in my parents was a bigger hurdle than a heart attack. I've done my best to myself and to Mum and Dad, and feel that I am worthy – and very appreciative – of this game I have played. This amazing, wondrous, not be dead for quids game of life.

EIGHT
ASK AND YOU MAY ... RECEIVE

I believe I have really seen God. Well, my version of whatever the next step is. Whatever happened to me the day I went to the beach and saw my grandparents, I believe a similar unexplainable, unquantifiable thing happened to me the day I had my heart attack.

It was a warm, April Sunday afternoon. I had left my flat to go for a walk. Walking down King William Road, I started sweating a bit too much and my back pack – which only had a water bottle in it – suddenly just got too heavy to carry. I had to take it off.

I was starting to get an uncomfortable, fretful, panicky feeling. It wasn't long before my heart felt like it was beating in my head and I was on the ground.

I said to myself: 'For fuck's sake, come on! Keep walking! Anyone would think you are having a heart attack!'

I was torn between trying to ignore what was going on (still thinking maybe I was having a panic attack) and turning around and walking home.

By the time I decided it was best to go home, I realised I didn't have the energy to do that. I felt sick, started vomiting

START WITH YOUR OWN ONION

and fell to the ground. Pain shot across my chest and down my arm and I realised that I was in deep trouble. There was no one around. Not a car had passed. I didn't have the strength to get my phone out of my bag. Suddenly, I became very weak. I realised I was going to die.

I looked up and saw a guy who lived in the same apartment block as me walking on the other side of the street. He had been over to my place many times. He suffered from depression, and it was particularly draining on my energy whenever he visited. He'd never bring over a packet of biscuits or bottle of milk – but would just arrive and expect my attention – which he got – and he got my counselling skills.

An unusual thing about Marty: he had an undetectable viral load for about 15 years, not needing to take medication in that time. His body just naturally suppressed the virus. I found it hard to deal with, considering the side effects I had had from the pills – that he had so much on his side, but he was still depressed. I was jealous, really. Not that I'm here to understand other peoples' actions, but he seemed to have most things going for him.

I was recently told he had a rather large member – and he was still depressed! If you are HIV positive, and you don't need to take medication due to your body's natural defences (so no side effects, no immune responses, no damage to your body from the virus), isn't that something to be happy about?

Anyway, I'm on the side of the road dying, and this guy on the other side of the road walked past me not even seeing me (I feel better if I believe that. I find it hard to believe that he would ignore me just because he was having a bad day) and I thought: *'Is this it? Dying on the side of the road in*

Adelaide? No! I haven't had the love of my life! I haven't done the travelling I want to do, I haven't won lotto!'

Then, I remember laughing and thinking *'Well if this is it, it has been good.'*

I looked up into the sky remembered all the faces I had seen in my life that had now gone to God. I looked at them all and said: 'I need help. Now!'

Within about 30 seconds, I looked over to see a woman closing her front gate and walking towards me with her dog on a lead. She had the look of *'Oh God, it's a junkie'* on her face until she got close to me and I asked her ever so politely: 'Excuse me please; could you ring an ambulance, please? I think I'm having a heart issue.'

She grabbed her phone and then a pair of hands lay on my shoulders and a young woman's face appeared to my left and said: 'Are you ok? I'm a nurse.' She took the phone from the other woman and started talking medical speak.

Then an elderly woman stood at my feet and said: 'Are you ok? I'm a retired doctor.'

I looked up into the sky and said: 'Thank you!'

The ambulance arrived. Again, two women got out, asked me questions. It wasn't long before I was thanking the women that had helped me, and I was at the hospital.

Doctors and nurses flustered about. About four or five times I was told 'Now, you know you are having a heart attack.' I was being wheeled into the surgery, and again I was asked 'Now you know you are having a heart attack?'

I replied: 'How the fuck can I be having a heart attack? I've never eaten McDonalds in my life!'

The team in the surgery all started to laugh and a woman leaned near me and said: 'Well darling, if you had have eaten McDonalds, you would have been here ten years ago.' She got me on that one.

I had visions of being cut wide open. The doctor told me that I was going to have a "procedure". I asked if he was going to cut me open. 'No,' was his reply. 'That's an operation. You are going to have a procedure.'

Not really knowing at the time what the difference was, he explained. A minor incision was made in my groin and I watched the rest on the screen. A balloon and a stent later and it was 4pm. Three hours since it began and I was in recovery.

A few days later, during my first shower, I had to take the bandage off expecting to find a big wound. As the water washed off the dried blood I could hardly see where they had entered my body. I'd scared myself to a point that I had to laugh. I was alive!

If I didn't know I was loved before, I certainly knew after. I had phone calls from all over the place enquiring as to my health. Mum and Dad came over to Adelaide and I will never forget seeing them both for the first time. After such an experience they really were the best thing. They sort of burst in the room, Mum rushed to me – tears and hugs and arms and kisses and *I love you*'s.

* * *

A great thing about being part of a big family is there are lots of people who can help with the workload when a family celebration rolls around. When I was working as a kitchen hand and apprentice I never attended any 18th or 21st birthdays because I was always working. When my sister Libby turned 40, I made a commitment that I was not going to miss any more big family celebrations.

Mum and Dad's turning of their decade parties and their 50th anniversary are some events that I have had a hand in organising, as well as the occasional no-particular-event family gatherings. Traditionally, I suppose, it's generally a matriarchal role cooking for these events. I have always enjoyed bucking trends.

It requires a lot of planning; from setting a date, locations, sending invitations (Libby's calligraphy skills always came in handy for these), guest lists, the menu, the children's table (when there were children – most are grown up by now), coffee and tea table, decorations, financing, setting up the space, and breaking it down at the end of the affair.

For Dad's 70th we made big banners that said "Happy Birthday!" and asked people to paint their hands and press them onto a large banner and sign their name. It was really great that Majella and her family, who were in the US, organised to send hand prints to add to the collection.

I was offered two jobs out of that occasion with celebrants who also did volunteer work with Dad. I told them, 'Sorry, this is a love job!'

Dad's 70th Birthday Menu
Spanakopitas (Spinach and Feta/Ricotta Triangles)
Oysters
Mini Pizzas
Chicken Sausage Rolls
Babaganoush and Avocado Dip with Turkish Bread
Olives
Fruit Platters
Sliced Ham and Flat Bread
Rare Roast Beef Wrapped in Blanched Lettuce Leaves with a Thai Dipping Sauce
Sushi Rolls
Chicken and Beef Skewers

Coffee, Tea and Milk
Chocolate Cake
Orange Cake
Sticky Date Pudding
Mince Pies
Pear Tarts
Chocolates Petit Fours
Cheesecakes
(And, of course) Birthday Cake

* * *

There were many speeches made in dedication to Dad – of which Paul's was full of laughter and poignancy. This was mine:

My Father Vincent Patrick Kelly is famous in Lismore, New South Wales – not that he has ever lived there, or even slept overnight. If truth be told, he has not got the highest opinion of it either.

But famous he is for a whistle stop tour he made nearly five years ago as a surprise guest for my 34th birthday. The time came for speeches and, 'Lo and behold!' Vinnie had one prepared, written by Margaret, that he delivered to 600 of my closest friends and to this day, whenever that party is mentioned,

"My Father and the Speech" are the first things remembered. It was the best party I will probably ever have.

As you may be are aware, I am rather unique in the Kelly family (no spouse, no children), but I believe I'm being true to the way God made me. I know that without Vin and Margie's love and support I wouldn't be here. When I revealed to Vinnie how God made me - with tears in his eyes, his words were:

'I don't care who you sleep with. You are still my son, and I love you.'

He has had to overcome major prejudices, both religious and social, to keep on loving his son. I know most of you here - and one might question yourselves - as to how you would cope with all that I've laid on them.

For about eight years whilst my brothers and sisters and spouses were setting up homes and having families, I lived through a war. I buried over 80 of my friends. I did not have a spouse or partner for comfort, but I feel I had someone better. My Mother and Father.

I don't know why I was touched so dramatically, but I do know I had the strength and hope of my parents.

We have become the best of friends as adults. As a child I felt my father was distant. However, as an adult, I realise what he must have had to go through to raise us all - and I totally forgive and understand him for that distance.

Vinnie has always been there for me - at one o'clock in the morning - picking me up at Candles restaurant, when I was a kitchen hand - or Springvale station, getting the last train home from work as an apprentice - or a shoulder to cry on when life seemed like it couldn't get any worse. The job of a parent is an extraordinary job and Vinnie has excelled.

He had no father in his life. As a child, the men that were in his life - from the stories I have heard - didn't seem to be all that flash as guardians. So without an example set, he has triumphed. I hope and pray that his example will keep, and be held dear to the following generations to come.

His taste in music has become so much better too, over the years! I feel I've done my bit to inspire him on that.

God knows none of us want to hear "Hooked On Classics" again!

Vinnie, I love you and I always will.

I also acknowledge I wouldn't be here, and he would only be half the man he is, without Margaret Josephine.

A Very Happy Birthday, Vincent x

* * *

Mum's Cheesecake

1 tin condensed milk
250gm cream cheese
Juice and zest of 3 lemons
1 packet of sweet biscuits shortbreads or Marie
50gm melted butter

- Crush biscuits and add melted butter
- Combine together and squash onto the base of a ring tin
- A light oiling of the side of the tin
- This mixture will fill a 25cm tin and give you a little left over
- Blend together milk, cheese, lemon and pour into tin
- Let this set in the fridge.

My version is to substitute cream cheese for mascarpone and add hazelnut meal to biscuit base with some cinnamon.

* * *

Baked Cheesecake

1kg of Neufchatel cheese
1 large lemon zest and juice
2 cups sugar
3 tablespoon flour
8 eggs – 5 whole and 3 yolks
Chosen crushed biscuit base (from Mum's Cheesecake recipe)

- First, organise a 20-25cm ring tin with the preferred base you would like to use
- Grease and flour the sides
- The options are quite varied – I have used a slice of cake to fit the tin or follow the previous recipe and to the base of crushed biscuit and melted butter. I've added toasted nuts or coconut or cocoa. It's your choice
- This can be done in a mix master or a food processor: add cream cheese and sugar together and lemon
- Add the flour and eggs make sure it is all well combined and there are no lumps on the side of the bowl
- Taste and make sure its lemony tart and sweet enough
- Bake at 230C for 10 minutes to get some colour
- Then go back to 130C for 1 hour
- Let set for 8 hours.

* * *

Auntie Bess's Sponge

This is the recipe given to me by Nana which Bess was famous for: her sponge. I think her version of a hot oven was still based on a wood fired stove. If a hot oven for you is a "flame thrower" and you think it may be too high, I wouldn't exceed 170C.

4 eggs
1 cup SR flour
1 cup plain flour
1 cup sugar
1 teaspoon of baking powder

- In a mix master, whip the eggs and sugar till light and fluffy
- Sift the flours together with the baking powder and fold it through the egg mix
- Bake in a hot oven for about 15 minutes.
- If you are making for a Swiss roll on a tray, keep your eye on it. It may not need 15 minutes if it's not that high
- If you are making a round tin it may take a little longer.

* * *

Auntie Shelia's Plain Cake
¼ lb butter
1 cup sugar
2 eggs
2 cups SR flour
1 cup milk

- Grease and flour your tin
- Cream the butter and sugar together till white

- Add 2 eggs
- Then add the flour and milk in small batches and mix well
- Bake in hot oven 450F (220 -230C) for 10 to 15 minutes.

* * *

Bread and Butter Pudding

Bread slices, enough to layer in a baking dish
10 eggs or yolks
150gm sugar
1L milk
Flavouring

- Combine eggs, sugar and milk
- Butter the bread and layer it in the dish you are making the pudding
- Between layers, literally anything can be added: berries, apples, pears, peaches, apricots, handfuls of chocolate buds or dried or candied fruits, jam or teaspoons of treacle or golden syrup (and don't forget a good splash of whiskey or brandy or even vodka)
- Once all the layers are done, pour the milk mixture into the dish, making sure the bread soaks up all the milk
- Sprinkle top with some sugar
- Bake in a moderate oven till brown and firm (this can be done in a bain-marie as well)
- This can be served hot straight from the dish or, once baked and set, it can be turned out onto a plate and served cold.

***

Citrus Tart

4 lemons
9 eggs
375gm sugar
300ml pure cream

- Zest and juice lemons
- For the base: use the recipe for pate sable line fluted flan dish, freeze then bake till light golden brown
- Combine eggs and sugar together
- Whisk cream lightly (don't whip it), then combine all ingredients together
- Into a prepared pre baked flan mould, pour your custard and then bake in a slow oven for about an hour to an hour and a half.

***

Lemon Butter

I do love this because it is very versatile. Its great on toast, it can be used with crepes or served with fruit. It takes a bit of work but then again: don't most good things?

5 lemons
450gm sugar
200gm butter
10 eggs

- In a stainless or ceramic bowl places on a pot of

hot water (best if it's not rapidly boiling), you can add all the ingredients and whisk till it thickens
- *Or* you can slowly add the mixture to the bowl and cook in smaller batches. Be careful as it can curdle quickly if you over-heat it!
- It is not far off ready when, with a whisk, the froth seems to "die down" and when you put a spoon in the mix it will appear thick on the back of the spoon
- If you put the spoon in as you start cooking, notice that hardly a trace will be left when you pull it out. When it is done it will be thick and coat the spoon nicely
- If it starts to look like it's got lumps in it, get it off the heat and cool it as soon as possible (possibly into a tray or container and into the freezer for a quick cool). You can cook the egg too much. *Never* boil it!

* * *

Lemon Delicious

60gm butter
¾ cup sugar
2 eggs, separated
4 tablespoons SR flour
1¼ cups milk
Zest and juice of one lemon

- Cream butter and sugar
- Add yolks, flour, grated rind and lemon juice
- Add milk

- Grease an oven proof casserole
- Cook in a bain-marie or moderate oven for 30 minutes

* * *

Mum's Nut Loaf

Mum used to make this when we were kids. She had special Nut loaf tins. They were a cylinder shape with lids on both ends. When cooked, they were a tube shape sliced into circles and buttered.

1 cup dates
½ cup sultanas
1 cup sugar
1 tablespoon butter
½ teaspoon salt
½ cup nuts, chopped
1 teaspoon of bi-carb soda
2 cups flour
1 egg
1 cup boiling water

- Chop the dates
- Combine with sultanas, sugar, butter and salt in a pot
- Add bi-carb soda and boiling water, mix well
- Add flour, nuts and egg, mix well
- Cook 350F for 50-60 minutes.

* * *

GREGORY KELLY

Mum's Pavlova

Originating with Margaret Fulton. This is a dessert that Mum excels in and I know she loves a piece too. Mum and I made a layered Pavlova for dads 80th birthday. I made about 6 other cakes but everyone lined up for the eight layered creation.

6 egg whites
2 cups castor sugar
1 teaspoon vanilla essence
1 teaspoon vinegar

- Whisk egg whites in a mix master and slowly add sugar
- Once all the sugar has been added it must be beaten for a while – at least 15-20 minutes
- All the sugar must be dissolved
- The essence and vinegar are to be folded in at the end
- Pop into a slow oven (130C) for a couple of hours
- After 2 hours, turn the oven off and leave the Pavlova in the oven till the oven is completely cold
- If making the day before, they can be left in the oven overnight
- Mum says the best result is baked in a combustion stove.

* * *

Nana Young's Fruit Cake

START WITH YOUR OWN ONION

1lb of seeded raisins
8oz chopped almonds
8oz glace cherries
8oz mixed peel
1 ½ lb sultanas
½ lb currants
2-3 cups brandy or orange juice
20oz plain flour
4oz SR flour
½ teaspoon salt
1 teaspoon grated nutmeg
1 teaspoon cinnamon
2 teaspoons mixed spice
1lb butter
1lb brown sugar
4 tablespoons marmalade or dark jam
2 teaspoons vanilla
8 eggs

- Marinate dried fruit and nuts in brandy or orange juice, preferably overnight
- Add the jam and spices to the fruit
- In a separate bowl cream the butter and sugar
- Add eggs
- Add cups full of fruit then flour alternately
- Making sure mixture is well combined before next addition
- This is a big cake made in the days when everyone ate fruitcake. Be aware that towards the end it may need to be transferred into a bigger bowl and finished mixing by hand
- I tend to line a 35 or 40cm tin with about 4 layers of paper between the tin and mixture. It's

in the oven for a long time and the paper protects the edges
- Bake in a moderate (150-175C) oven for about 4 hours
- Nana Young made this by hand most of her life. As fruit cake isn't as popular as it once was, I have a collection of tins – 10 and 15cm sizes – which I used for this mixture. I generally get at least 6 or 7 cakes which tend to take about an hour and a half to two hours to cook.

***

Fruit Mince

I do have a thing about certain Christmas treats and these are one of them. I use pate sable as the base for the pies and they are delicious.

240gm suet
240gm apples, dried (I have also used fresh grated apple which works well)
240gm sultanas
240gm currants
240gms raisins
240gm chopped peel
240gm sugar
8gm mixed spice
30gm mixed almonds
150ml rum, brandy, or sugar syrup

- Make sure all fruit if too big is chopped up well

- Combine all ingredients and let stand for at least two weeks.

Today you can just buy a packet of suet, so just be aware that it has flour in it. Fresh suet is just a fat so it is a little different.

* * *

Panforte or Sienna Cake
4 cups almonds
4 cups hazelnuts
250gm dates
250gm dried apricots
250gm dried pears
250gm crystallised ginger (chopped fine)
2 cups plain flour
¾ cup cocoa
1 dessertspoon nutmeg
1 tablespoon cinnamon
2 dessertspoons mixed spice
1 teaspoon ground ginger
2 cups sugar
2 cups honey

- Roast nuts
- Roughly chop the fruit and ginger (if you don't like big blasts of ginger then chop this as fine as you can)
- Mix dry ingredients all together thoroughly
- Using a candy thermometer, boil honey and sugar till soft ball stage (if you don't have one then for about 5 minutes)

- Beware! This is hot!
- Pour honey mix onto the dry ingredients. It will start to go firm so you must act quickly
- Onto a tray that has been lined with edible rice paper, pop in a moderate oven for 30 minutes
- Let it cool on a rack and store in an airtight container
- This is something that will last for a long time and gets better with age.

* * *

Middle Eastern Orange Cake

This cake was a constant at the Queenscliff Hotel and over the years I have made many variations using different nut meals and certain fruits like mandarins or peaches. Essentially, if using different fruit, it's got to resemble the same volume as the oranges.

2 large oranges
½ lb of almond meal
½ lb of caster sugar
6 eggs

- Boil the oranges for a good 20 minutes three times and replace the water each time. This is to get rid of the bitterness in the pith
- Once that's done, let them cool
- Discard the part where it was connected to the tree and any pips
- Puree the flesh and skin together
- Add eggs and meal and sugar to the puree

- Grease and flour or line a 25cm ring tin with baking paper
- Bake in a moderate oven till firm in the centre and coloured.

* * *

Fig and Pecan Pie

This is one of the easier simple baked goods. It's not really a pie and I'm not sure why it was called that! Its great served with a plain yoghurt or crème fraiche.

250gm dried chopped figs
250gm pecans
3 egg whites
250gm brown sugar

- Whip eggwhites and add sugar
- Add chopped figs and pecans
- Line a 30cm ring tin with baking paper
- Bake in a moderate oven for about ½ hour
- Skewer the centre to see if cooked. It can go for another 15 minutes or so in the oven
- Let it cool in the tin.

* * *

Apricot Tofu Cake

Base
1 cup rice flour
1 cup fine desiccated coconut
1 tablespoon pear concentrate to sweeten

100gm Nuttelex or vegetarian type fat to make moist

- Combine all ingredients
- Press into a 30cm (lined with baking paper) ring tin.

Filling

375gm of tofu
500ml soy milk
1 ½ cups of coconut
250gm dried apricots – boiled in water to soften and left to cool before using
1-2 tablespoons of pear concentrate to sweeten

- Add tofu into food processor first and blend
- Add all other filling ingredients
- Taste and check for sweetness
- Pour onto base and bake in a moderate oven till set. About an hour
- Let cool in the tin.

* * *

Sticky Date Pudding
1 cup chopped dates
1 cup milk
½ cup sugar
3 tablespoons butter
1 teaspoon bicarb of soda
1 cup SR flour

- Boil dates, milk, sugar and butter
- Stir in bicarb of soda. Take off heat and let cool
- Then add flour and mix well till all lumps have been beaten out
- Grease and flour baking tin (8")
- Place mixture in tin and cover with foil
- Bake in a moderate oven 350F (180-200C)
- You can bake in a bain-marie (large baking dish ½ filled with hot water) for about ¾ of an hour
- To test if cake is baked insert a skewer into centre or lightly push in the centre and if it springs back cake is done.

* * *

Summer Pudding

Use an assortment of mixed berries, depending on the size of your bowl and how many people you are going to serve. Approx 1kg of berries should do about 8 people

½ loaf of day-old bread slices (enough to line the bowl you're using)
1kg mixed berries
150-200gm caster sugar
100gm butter

- You can use 500gm of mixed frozen berries and a couple of punnets of strawberries
- These are then cooked quickly in about a tablespoon of butter
- When it comes to a boil add sugar to sweeten taste

- Then, take off heat and pour through a strainer
- Using day-old bread that has had the crusts removed, quickly soak the bread in the juice
- Line the bowl overlapping the rim (soaked bread needs to form a seal)
- Then put berries in the bowl and line the top with bread (as done with the sides)
- Cover with glad wrap and place a weight onto the top (try not to over press the pudding)
- Let it set and chill for 4 to 5 hours, but preferably overnight
- Turn out and use the excess liquid as a sauce and serve with cream.

NINE
CELEBRATE – IT'S EASY

Food can incite passion and drama – and that can be great if the company is dull! I prefer the people I share a table with to have more to say than the food. A passionate – and a bit dramatic – company makes for lively debate and some great storytelling.

Fortunately I have shared many life-affirming, fabulous moments over a meal. I always say I love every meal that someone else has made for me.

I've had private dinner parties, catered for family celebrations and events, and amazing services at work where everything goes flawlessly. These are very rare. I'm a bit hard on myself sometimes, but I know and appreciate when something goes really well. I'm referring to when all expectations are surpassed, and incredible memories are made. You know when it is special.

My 34th birthday party at the Winsome with 600 (of my closest friends) was such an event. There were eight DJ's, a sound system, a jazz band, volunteers who helped with the food, fireworks, light shows, *five* birthday cakes, male, female and transgender performance artists – all donated skills and services for the night. We raised $1500 for local HIV issues and premiered the Winsome Hotel as a GLBTIQ, everyone's safe place. We converted it from a country and western pub where there were fights most nights, to a place where even older ladies came and had an afternoon sherry on the veranda.

* * *

Wherever I have lived I do enjoy a dinner party, and Punt Road holds a few special memories. It was a bit of an awkward, pokey little flat, but with a redesign of furnishings I turned the small space into a room big enough for a dinner for 16 people. This number of people was only done once! I sent out invites and received a full complement of acceptances. I just love when people put a bit of thought into a letter, reply or speech. It helps cement the event and adds to the occasion.

Too often I find people don't have enough practice at speaking off the cuff or with a prepared speech, and it's only at funerals that, without too much practice, people are forced to speak about their loved ones.

Birthday parties without a toast to acknowledge the achievement of getting to the age that is being celebrated, no acknowledgement to the host or thanks to the guests or any formality can be a bit dull and anti-climactic.

After a warm speech I always notice a certain deeper bonding of the group involved. This point is also the time at a party that some guests can exit and some kick on. I find it an important part of an event. People might quietly want to leave, but at least stay for the speeches and the cake and then can go.

One response to the dinner for 16 at Punt Road was on

the letterhead of a law firm. I remember opening it and my first thought was: *'What have I done wrong?'* I realised as I read there was nothing wrong! It read:

Dear Mr Kelly,
   "Unauthorised Abuse of Party Privilege"
   It has come to our attention that the inhabitants of your residence proposed to indulge in feasting (to the extent of 15 courses no less), ribaldry and excessive consumption on the evening of 28 July 1991.
   Purely temporal considerations have allowed the matter to remain unattended to so far, however, this in no way prejudices our client's right in this matter.
   Our client wishes us to inform you that she will not tolerate an evening's entertainment of the abovementioned magnitude without her express consent or authorisation, necessitating her presence on 28 July 1991 at the premises of 555 Punt Rd, South Yarra.
   Our client who is conducting a business negotiations in Sydney that weekend wrapping up a squillion dollar deal, will be required to return specially for the event in her private Lear jet, consequently, she may be slightly late. Do not, however, take this as a sign that these proceedings are to be regarded lightly. We assure you of the seriousness of our client's intentions.
   We look forward to your reply, which we expect to be delivered on the night of 28 July 1991.

Yours faithfully,
   Bronwyn

. . .

My apartment wasn't very big so I made the bedroom at the front the smoking (which was obviously still fashionable) and nibbles room. I pushed the bed against the wall, the couch went into the bedroom, and the dinner table and chairs for 16 just made it in the lounge room.

As everyone arrived, they were escorted into the front room and I served a lemon verbena punch with vodka with Nori rolls, prosciutto and grissini, sundried olives, roasted soy sauce, and ginger mixed nuts.

As I was going to heat the entree, the gas simply went off. There was no gas going into the pipes. I rang the gas company, and was told someone would come that evening.

I was slightly hysterical, and said: 'I have 16 people for dinner, I need the gas now!'

Maybe that helped, maybe it didn't!

I ran down the back stairs and knocked on the apartment door below me, explained my predicament and asked to borrow their kitchen. They were very gracious, and let me use it.

The entrée was a pasta bon-bon, with a filling of ham, carrot, celery, onion, mushroom and sweet potato. The sheets of pasta I made had green and red fettuccini stripes, and were shaped in a bon-bon, with chives pulling the ends together. They were already prepared and just needed heating up, to be served in a bowl of a rich chicken and tomato broth. I walked up two flights of stairs with the heated food and Joanne and Suzanne served the guests.

The main was a Chicken Thai Curry – which, again, was cooked and just needed heating through. By this stage, all I needed to do was stir-fry the vegetables and cook the rice. These were served in bowls, and I let everyone help themselves.

During the serving of the main, the gas man arrived! He

started tapping away at the pipes. I can't remember what had happened, but by the time the main course was finished, the gas was fixed! This did cause some anxious moments but also some funny ones too. One deals with each situation as it arises – it seems easier that way.

I always think that it's important to mark an event with a short speech of recognition. Just to point out that that moment – whatever it was – would never happen again. It was highly unlikely that those 16 people would ever be in the same room again. As it is, several people who were at that dinner have since passed away, so it will never happen again.

Jim Scarlett was such a man to rise to the challenge of a speech, he dedicated this to me:

Prandium Dandium Est,
Being a short burst of Eloquence written
In Praise of Gregory V Kelly
Host extraordinaire

What's in the envelope written so beautifully?
An invite to Gregory's –dinner tonight
The mouth is awash with fluids digestative,
A vision of dinner with soft candle light

"Yes I shall come" I cry through the telephone,
"Rings on my fingers and bells on my toes;
"Bottle of wine, vintage delectable;
"Not only these: I'll put on my best clothes"

Room very beautiful- look at those cornices
Painted pure white by a craftsman, no doubt.

GREGORY KELLY

Walls were replastered prior to undercoat; then
Painted pale blue the apartment throughout.

Sixteen are invited, friends all of Gregory's
We are all honoured to share at his board
Eat his creations of dainty comestibles.
Tippling the wine when it's gone, more is poured

Canapés, pasta and chicken we (curried) have
The food: it is splendid, the company, gay.
We will remember this banquet superlative,
We shan't forget it before judgement day.

For it's a foretaste of all things celestial;
Precursor, it is of the feasting on high:
Feast Dionysian, revel of Bacchus,
Communion or love feast way up in the sky.

Gregory: friend, chef extraordinary,
Organised this for his friends – you and me.
Credit to him for this celebration
For he's the creator of all our glee.

Charge now your tumblers, all of my auditors;
Charge them and raise them up now for a toast:
To Gregory Kelly- all of us love you;
We drink to your health now, good friend and host

Oronsay Goodthwack
28th July 1991

* * *

START WITH YOUR OWN ONION

It was a truly remarkable speech, which I was incredibly proud to hear. A great touch was it being served with David's (my brother in law) home brew.

The dessert was a slice of Chocolate Marquis with cream and mandarins slightly frozen in brandy and passionfruit.

Soft cheeses followed – Mascarpone and Stracchino – with quince paste and fruit bread.

Coffee and petit fours – nut chocolate clusters, slices of Sienna cake, chocolate wafers, and brandied cumquats (which were so tart they were almost unpalatable - but had a huge kick!).

Libby and David, Joanne and Matt, Bronwyn Ross, Neville, Jim, Susanne, Adrian, Doug, Helen, Michelle and Ducca and myself plus another (I think there was an apology on the night).

* * *

An event happened on Punt Rd in 1986. It didn't start out as an event but it became one! It was my tree-trimming party at Christmas. Not that I've had many of late, but the ones I've had have been memorable. The idea is that everyone brings a decoration, preferably handmade, for the Christmas tree, and a non-perishable food item is placed under the tree to be given to a charity.

I was at home drinking gin and putting up the Christmas tree, feeling a bit sad and tragic doing it by myself. There was a knock on the door, followed by another a few minutes later, and within about an hour I had about ten people in my home. They saw the light on and decided to drop in.

I went from a bit sad and lonely to, an hour later, having

a party on my hands! I was told the tree looked sad and that it needed a makeover. It truly was a spontaneous night, and when it was over, in the wee small hours before dawn, I had an amazing tree.

It was one of those moments you're not sure what happened, or how – other than just pure fabulousness. I decided the next year that I would supply the tree and I had decorations, but people got into making things that sparkled! Bags of sugar, tins of tomatoes, toothpaste, women's hygiene things – all sorts of kitchen and personal items were brought along. There had been bush fires over the time so the goods were donated to the communities affected.

One tree-trimming in Byron in about 1995 was quite amazing. At the time, Shane and I lived in a two-level apartment and so the tree was able to be about four metres high.

About 150 people were treated to performances of the Christmas fairies Scott and Steven, beautiful music by Terri (Mrs T), great food and good times. We gave four carloads of goods to the CWA intended for people affected by the drought.

I have only had one or two tree-trimmings in Adelaide. Basically, I haven't been around at Christmas time – but I donated all the goods from those events to the *Positive Living Centre*, which had a pantry for people who are HIV positive on low incomes.

It's an idea that I wish would catch on. Instead of going to a party and expecting to be entertained, the guest brings the reason to be part of a party. A special thing about the North Coast was that the entertainment came with those invited. I developed an expression for Adelaide: 'In Byron, all you had to do was whisper in someone's ear *I'm having a party,* and 200 people will show up. In

Adelaide, you have to give 200 head jobs to get 20 people to show up!'

It took some time to get used to the different dynamics of throwing a party in Adelaide. I have a tendency to over-cater a bit, but when 50 people say they are coming and 15 show up, I took that as a personal slur. It took going to a few other peoples' parties to realise that it wasn't just me! This happened to the "A" gays as well!

The only thing that I can think of is that the North Coast events were few and far between. So when one happened, it was an occasion that everyone wanted to get in on. Maybe Adelaide is big enough that there is a chance something else might come along that might be better. So one keeps guard, if one is going to an event, or not – just in case! I don't know. For whatever reason, it's a bitch for catering.

Sometimes when I have catered for events I leave some things intentionally left part done. If I don't get to serve them, then they can have a second life at some other event. If I buy salmon that isn't used – it becomes a rillettes, cheese can be frozen in small cubes and used for an omelette; even fruit can be frozen and used in smoothies – that sort of thing. I hate waste of any sort.

Dinner parties for me can be lots of fun. Most of the time, people on the North Coast are prepared to stay the night due to travelling distances and drinking. One such party in Byron was a highlight for me. Again, at Wollumbin Street, Shane and I prepared the food, and Shane and his partner at the time did the "tzushing".

We draped Bougainvillea on the curtain rod and attached it to the balustrade above the table. Blue velvet drapes just appeared and other bits and pieces were placed around to make the event visually spectacular. The meal was pretty good too! Prawns with a spinach salad, and whole baked snapper with a herb puree, which Shane ever-so-elegantly pulled apart and served up. There was a polenta bake with tapenade, a capsicum salsa and a vegetable curry in a coconut milk sauce with steamed rice, potato salad, and for dessert, a baked cheesecake with a raspberry coulis.

Many of the memorable moments in my adult life have a close connection with food and Shane; our friendship makes an event. We have always bantered against each other, laughing uncontrollably and that laughter is infectious. He had so much hospitality experience as well as an ingrained creativity he could turn the most humble of areas into some special place, thus giving that area his blessing. I was probably the one to fret at big events, but Shane, through his leadership and dynamic sense of occasion, almost forced me (willingly) to enjoy these moments; these gatherings of people; these opportunities to experience life's greatest gift: our loved ones.

* * *

Tapenade
Combine:
200gm of pitted olives
Several cloves of garlic
A few sprigs of rosemary and thyme
A splash of balsamic vinegar (enough to wet the olives)
Fresh cracked pepper
6 anchovies
A dessertspoon of Dijon mustard
A little oil

- Blitz in a food processor till fine paste

* * *

Hommos (Hummus, Hommus – whatever!)
Chickpeas
Lemon juice
Tahini (¼ tahini to ¾ chickpeas)
Salt and pepper
Garlic, crushed

- Dried chickpeas soaked overnight in salted water, boiled till soft, or you can use tins of cooked chickpeas, or if you have a pressure cooker, cook in one of those and keep the liquid as it's the best vegetable stock ever. A rich nutty lovely flavour
- Boil till soft and then mash fine (but can be chunky)
- Add enough lemon juice to taste (ratio 1 can = 1 lemon)
- Tahini – about ¼ tahini to ¾ chickpeas
- Add the crushed garlic and salt and pepper

I have used mayonnaise instead of tahini and rough chopped parsley, mint, spring onions and oregano.

* * *

My Babaganoush
2 large eggplants
4 cloves of garlic roasted with eggplant
3 lemons juice and zest

1 cup olive oil
1 large bunch of basil

- Halve eggplants, score the flesh deeply but not through to the skin
- Salt liberally and let stand for at least half an hour, then wash thoroughly
- Coat with oil and roast in a hot oven till soft
- Blend roasted pulp in a food processor
- With processor on add roasted garlic, lemon juice
- Basil and slowly pour in the oil as its processing
- When all combined and smooth add salt and pepper.

* * *

Salmon Rillettes

500gm salmon
1 cup fish stock
250gm butter
3 tablespoons of oil
Salt and pepper
Chopped fennel

- Poach salmon in stock for about 5 minutes
- Set aside let cool
- Process quickly with oil and butter
- Season and add chopped herbs
- Place in small bowls let set or roll into tubes in gladwrap then foil. This can be done in small batches and frozen.

* * *

Samosa Filling

2kg cubed potatoes
200gm butter
5 onions
6 sprigs parsley
6 sprigs mint
30gm curry powder
1 tablespoon cumin
1 tablespoon powdered coriander
1 tablespoon ginger
1 tablespoon cinnamon
1 teaspoon turmeric
1 teaspoon paprika
2 cups of peas

- Boil peeled potatoes till soft but not mushy. I tend to add the peas at this stage before the potatoes are done to save on washing up
- Sauté onions and add spices
- Combine all together
- Add salt and pepper
- Let cool before using with pastry.

* * *

Samosa Pastry

1 ½ cup plain flour
¾ teaspoon salt
1 tablespoon of oil or ghee
½ cup warm water

- Mix flour and salt together
- Add oil and water mix the flour forming a ball
- Mix may need to add a little more water
- When the ball is firm and all the flour is combined, a 10 minute knead is good then a ½ hour rest before use
- Roll out to desired thickness and make samosa
- They can be fried or baked, I prefer them baked.

* * *

Mussels

1kg mussels
1 large onion
50gm butter
2 cups white wine

- Sauté the onions in the butter till clear
- Add the mussels
- Herbs and wine
- Cover with a damp cloth
- Steam the mussels for a few minutes
- When most look like they have opened give them a stir and drain
- Discard those that don't open
- Serve straight away or they can be let to go cold and eaten. Great as an entrée or appetiser.

* * *

Provencal Soup

(One of my favourite soups)

5 chopped onions
10 red capsicums
5-6 sticks of celery
5 carrots
2 tablespoons tomato paste
6 cardamom pods
2 tablespoons of ground coriander
4 teaspoons of ground cumin
Lots of garlic
Bay leaves
Fish stock, 2 or 3 litres

- Sauté onions till clear
- Add garlic and then chopped capsicums
- Add chopped carrots and celery
- Add spices then fish stock
- Boil till all vegies are soft
- Puree, add salt and pepper, lemon juice to taste
- It's really good with a splash of Pernod
- I prefer to serve this with a dollop of aioli.

* * *

Avocado and Roesti Salad

- Make roesti by boiling potatoes the day before in their skins till they are able to be pierced with a knife
- Next day peel and grate on a grater (large hole) add a bit of garlic and salt and pepper
- Shape together to form discs
- Coat in flour

- Then fry in oil till brown both sides and can then put in the oven
- When really crispy spread the roesti with tapenade
- Chop some iceberg lettuce
- Place on top
- Fan avocado place on top of lettuce
- A simple vinaigrette or something a bit more lavish a mayonnaise type dressing goes well
- And some chopped tomato
- Sprinkle with chopped spring onions as well.

* * *

My dear friend Thora Tutty was close to celebrating her 80th birthday. I had checked with Thora if her family had plans to celebrate. They didn't, so I asked Thora if I could arrange something special, what would she like. She decided upon a sit down lunch. The next task was to find out what foods she wanted. Robyn, Thora's daughter, and I questioned Thora about what foods she liked and we sat down and started to organise. We invited help from Shane and Neil, and another friend Tony. They prepared food and the wonderful displays of roses that decorated the house and dinner tables. They cooked and served the guests and were guests themselves. We invited Thora's best friend, Ruby, and Thora's other daughters and their husbands. I also took the opportunity – as it was close to Mum's birthday – to give Mum and Dad a plane fare, and got them up for the event. Unfortunately, all of Thora's sons-in-law declined the invite to attend. They, according to Thora, couldn't deal with the "poof" thing!

One of the greatest compliments I've ever heard (that I

will take a little credit for) was primarily directed at Shane and was from Ruby. She told Shane – in a most expressive way – that Thora's 80th Birthday lunch was the greatest meal she had ever had in her life. People often throw out superlatives; some are sincere – a lot are not. The look on Ruby's face that day said it all; pure sincerity came from her words and eyes.

I remember Thora being in rapture! She loved oysters, so we had a few different varieties of those. We had bisque made from local yabbies, baked salmon, and a chocolate beetroot cake. It truly was a fantastic day.

My dedication to Thora:

"Ladies and Gentlemen

I remember the first time I met Thora about 8 years ago.

I had a friend up from Sydney and we had just got out of the car, after hitting the hill at the Main Arm address. (A long steep incline that a lot of people refused to drive)

I looked at Thora and said "You drive that hill?" She smiled and said of course!

I thought something was special about this girl!

Then we sat down to an Asian banquet I knew something was special. It is a very rare thing for a woman of her age to cross cultures when it comes to cooking.

Since then, and thanks to Mr Piccles (who bought the house next door to Thora and Robyn which I rented), I had the pleasure of having HRH The Queen and The Princess as my neighbours in the Queendom of Dunoon. A fabulous time of planting and coming home to find my clothes taken off the line folded and home cooked meals and of course "Have you got a singlet on?" (Thora's major concern)

GREGORY KELLY

My first impression of Thora Tutty was of a very special woman.

I would only change that statement to say Thora is a special angel. An angel I'm honoured to call a friend.

Whether you are mother, daughter, father or son - the most important thing is I feel to have is friendship.

I'm humbled to have in one space, at one time, a group of very special friends who literally, have brought me back from "The Other Side" on more than one occasion. I cannot express gratitude enough. And so we are here for a reason -

Please charge your glasses, and toast Thora Tutty! A very happy birthday!

TEN
KNOW YOUR COUNTRY

2⁰⁰²   I was at a loose end in Byron. Everything was far away, and with little money to buy petrol, getting from one place to another was tedious. A couple of events occurred around the same time:

One) my landlord – who was one of the biggest crooks in the area – had asked for a rent increase, *again*. I had not even signed the lease and he upped the rent. He first said rent would be $65 a week and he was going to open a little take-away, which I was going to run, right on Tallow's beach. Anyway, that didn't happen.

We agreed on $65, but as I was signing the contract he said, 'Oh, I have to put it up to $80.' That was still within my price range and so I begrudgingly agreed. Within a month, instead of fortnightly rent he wanted calendar-monthly rent. The next month he wanted $100 a week. Each month, for about six months of the lease, there was some other financial screw.

I gave two weeks' notice in the last two weeks of my lease. He said I needed to give him a month notice as we had agreed that I pay monthly. I reminded him that I had not agreed to anything. It was he who changed the rules.

I drew his attention to the original terms on the lease and told him that he had broken the terms at least five times. I started to realise that living in a beautiful spot (which it certainly was along the Coolamon Scenic route) didn't mean a thing if it had no respect or love.

Two) I was at the beach at Broken Head and a cry came out on the beach, alerting everyone that cars were being trashed. I ran up to the car park – which is a decent ascent – to find that my car and about five others had every window smashed. Trying to get a signal on a mobile to ring police was difficult. When we finally did get in touch with police, we were told that a police car wouldn't come out and we had to drive the cars to the police station. It was a difficult trip, as I only had half a windscreen, which was not made any better by being told: 'Just kids probably. Yeah, well, you were at Kings Beach. There's not much we can do.'

And they were true to their word, nothing happened! Oh, and the cars were unroadworthy and weren't allowed to be driven away again.

Three) A few days after the car incident, a friend of mine was made homeless because his flat mates had found out he was HIV positive. He came home to find all of his stuff on the street and the locks changed. This sort of stuff was supposed to happen elsewhere. This was Byron: peace, love and hippies. I lost the love for Byron.

* * *

Two girlfriends of mine had moved to South Australia and sent out an invite to come and help them on the farm and in their pub. So, in 2003, I moved to some of the hardest country I had ever seen in my life. The Mallee is harsh and unforgiving country, right on the edge of the desert. The farm was in a little place not really a town. I learnt how to drive a tractor, bleed its engine, and all sorts of farm things I picked up along the way.

It was the total opposite of Byron with its lush green hills – this place was sandy, low desert, sheep, wheat, potato and canola country. I did enjoy the farm, but eight months was enough.

I remember spending about three days digging up a hideous weed with big thorns called Calthrop. Not the most stimulating job in the world. I looked up to the sky and said: 'It's got to be better than this!'

Within two weeks I found a course I wanted to do in Adelaide and found out about a gay men's housing co-op. I applied for the co-op and was offered a choice of a two bedroom apartment close to town or a three bedroom house in the suburbs. I remember driving further and further away from the city and saying to Grant that I didn't care if it had a swimming pool, I wanted the apartment. I got accepted for the course and moved into the apartment in the same week.

* * *

Adelaide has been very good to me. Studying, volunteering at a little theatre in town, radio presenting, stage work, HIV health promotion, acting in a health advertisement that has been shown at many of the film nights, meeting Grant and having him help me do projects of furniture restoration have all been highlights.

I had a collection of dead peoples' stuff in different stages of disrepair. After many hours in the shed, I have my own furniture that I have rebuilt with Grant's assistance.

In many respects, I arrived in Adelaide a sickly fellow with bad teeth and my possessions were basically a bit crap. Now, I have great teeth (and, therefore, good health) thanks to Dr Liz Coates, Margie Steffens and the team at the Adelaide Dental Hospital. Also, I have some great furniture that I have made or rebuilt, including my wonderful bed.

* * *

Curing Olives

- Large olives need to be scored (cut not all the way through) down the side of the olive. If they are small olives, like wild olives, they don't need to be scored.
- Make sure to pick through the olives and make sure they are clean and free from stems.
- Depending on the volume of olives you have, I tend to have enough for a 10 litre bucket. As a guide, I dissolve at least a cup and a half of salt into some hot water then half-fill the bucket with cool water. I then taste to make sure it's salty enough. This means that it's unpalatable, but it needs to be. I like to make sure that there's enough salt to kill any germs and no chance of any fermenting happening.
- When the brine is completely cool, add the scored olives and cover. I like to make sure all are submerged by weighting something over them.
- The first brine I leave for about three or four days. I leave each new brine for about five or six

- days, and then repeat the process. Empty the brine, make new brine and soak olives.
- I've done this for about four or five weeks. I have checked other recipes and I may do a bit of overkill, but I do like to make sure that no living bug can thrive! When I'm satisfied that they are tasty I add peppercorns, bay leaves, lemon peel, garlic, maybe some sticks of rosemary and thyme to the end brine.
- Then, they can be left in the bucket with a lid, or I tend to put them into large jars with a tight lid. I pour about 1 ½ cm of olive oil on top of the brine and make sure all the olives are below the line of oil.
- It is really important at this stage to use sterilised spoons, tongs, jars and to wash the buckets after each stage with hot soapy water.
- Over a period of time, mould can appear on the top of the liquid. Apparently this is a good thing for some people as it is a seal. It can be removed easily with no apparent damage to the olives. Once the jars are opened, I tend to keep them in the fridge.
- If you are unsure as to the saltiness of your brine, I was told by Mr Kostoglou that if you float an egg in the brine that part of the egg should jut out of the water with the diameter of a twenty cent piece. If you've got that then your brine is salty enough.

* * *

Popcorn and Mixed Nut Brittle

1 ½ cup nuts
1 cup coarse crumbled popcorn
1 ½ cups sugar
½ cup corn syrup
1/3 cup water
3 tablespoons butter
1 teaspoon salt
¼ teaspoon baking soda (bi carb)
1 teaspoon vanilla

- Lightly roast the nuts in the oven
- Mix with popcorn when cool
- Bring sugar, corn syrup, and water to boil
- Add a teaspoon of lemon juice and alcohol (spirit)
- Cook the candy till it reaches 310F on a candy thermometer
- Remove from heat
- Stir in the salt, bi carbonate of soda and vanilla
- Add nuts and popcorn and quickly stir all together
- Spread onto a tray with baking paper on it and press the top with another sheet of baking paper to spread the brittle out evenly
- When it starts to cool, quickly cut with a knife with a lightly-oiled blade. Repeat light oiling after two or three slices.
- Let it set and don't eat too much in one go!
- I have found that this recipe will take three or four cups of popcorn and double nuts and seeds can be added
- Great for pepitas, sesame, sunflower, puffed rice any dry nut

- Don't use dried fruit, because that will dissolve the toffee, so it's not a good mix
- Dipped in chocolate is pretty fabulous
- Store in several air tight containers so you don't have to expose the entire batch to the constant opening and reopening!

* * *

Adelaide has enabled me tap into lots of creativity; singing, making short movies, a bit of acting, radio, volunteering at a little theatre in town, performing at the Bear events and, of course, the study. I thoroughly enjoyed the Certificate III in Community Services, as well as two Diplomas in Community Welfare; one in Mental Health, the other in Counselling Skills.

I loved meeting new people from totally different lives. People who came to Australia as refugees, people living with major physical disabilities or mental health issues, stricter Christian (or religious types), single mothers, young people, older people looking for something different in their lives. In a great way, they all touched me profoundly. There's something to be said for a classroom environment where the objective of some of the classes in counselling is to bare a bit of your soul, and having enough trust in the lecturers and students to do that.

I believe if you are born in this country – even at the lowest socio economic level – there is some fragile safety net. Nothing can compare to the stories of people who are living peacefully one day, to having to run with nothing but what they have with them at that moment. Imagine leaving family, country, home and belongings because you have just seen your mother, father and other family members raped and shot. Not just you, but everyone around running for their lives.

Can you conceive being in the middle of a dentist appointment, having a root canal treatment, and half way through drilling, when it's at the exposed nerve, bullets start flying above your head. Everyone has to run to the jungle to hide and for the next eight years and two refugee camps, that hole in your tooth is still exposed?

Can you imagine being able to get your six children safely to the refugee camps, but your husband was shot before leaving the country, then watching four of your children die in the camps to be buried with others without too much ceremony – no space for personal grief?

Can you conceive being chained on the back of a truck being transported from refugee camps in one country to the next? Can you conceive watching a child with an AK 47 pointing at your mother whilst that child feels your mother's breast?

In social situations, when someone has a blanket belief about the refugee situation, I like to challenge some preconceived notions with some of the truths that I've been told. (I think mainly because I'm a bit of a shit stirrer! Also, I know life just isn't black or white – a lot of people who believe in white have never tried to appreciate the black ...)

Imagine leaving or escaping to another country and telling no one, because if you did, they could inform the secret police? The decision would have to be based on never being able to tell loved ones where you're going as it would be jeopardising their lives. Based on this same premise, you would have to make a decision that you may never hear from or see your loved ones again.

I have had the utmost privilege to have met such people

who have been through the experiences I've just mentioned.

My dear friend Augustina is from Liberia. She has been a source of delight and strength considering the extremes of humanity that she has been through in her life. Along with Peg and Victoria, we all met at Port Adelaide TAFE whilst studying. We've all been out with Augustina to different gatherings like birthdays and funerals, independence or national country days, celebrations of different countries and other celebratory events.

The greatest compliment I ever received was during a celebration of Liberian National Day. Augustina invited me and two other friends to the event, during which she asked me, 'Greg, can you dance?'

The music was a groovy reggae percussion sound and I said, 'Sure, I can dance.' We were dancing away and I started to notice a group of women in the front row of the pews – dressed immaculately in matching sarong-type traditional outfits with amazing head wear. They seemed to be pointing and talking in my general direction. There was obviously some lively discussion.

I also noticed a group of young boys and men, maybe 15 to 25 years old, that were starting to congregate in the corner. They were pointing and looking in my general direction.

I started thinking possibly my pants were split, something was on my face, I'd done something wrong, or was still doing something wrong. Something was going on! After a while, Augustina said that she needed to go out for a cigarette and I followed. She said to me: 'Well, Gregory, you got that room talking!' in her expressive style.

'What have I done? Is it bad? I saw people pointing. What have I done wrong?'

'No one in that room thought a white boy could dance and, boy, YOU can dance! You got those hips swaying. You know about rhythm. The people say to me, "Augustina, you've taught that white boy to dance."' She said that she told them she had not taught me – that she was shocked as them.

I burst out laughing and I must admit I was bloody thrilled that about 200 beautifully dressed, gorgeous black people think that I had rhythm!

Augustina calls me her white brother. A title I cherish.

I did my placement (needed for the Diplomas) at a Community centre in Ottoway run by Kathy, another girlfriend met through study. I was privileged to be able to organise a Liberian cooking class, with Augustina running the class. It was great. She took me to shops I never knew existed and would never have found on my own. It was funny, we'd go into a shop and the customers would be all African or Middle Eastern, mainly women; some in groups, some with husbands and Augustina and me walking around as she explained different ingredients to me.

Another cooking highlight I had at the Community Centre was an anti-poverty celebration lunch – we involved as many community members as possible. A lot of the people that came to the centre had issues of a physical and or mental health nature. One such person was Pam, who one day left what she was doing with her family, leaving her comfortable world, and slept rough. She had major mental health issues; she was very shy and talked about ending her life many times. Part of the community event was an op shop fashion parade. We took ten regulars from the centre to the large op shop close by and they picked two or three outfits to be part of the parade. Pam was really excited by the event and it seemed she really enjoyed herself. A few

START WITH YOUR OWN ONION

weeks later, Pam lay on the railway tracks and a train cut off her leg. She was trying to leave this planet.

We had 90 guests at the event and about eight women had volunteered to help me cook and work the kitchen. I was making a simple pumpkin soup, a chicken breast wrapped in bacon with a cream sauce, roast potatoes, steamed vegies, and a plum pudding dessert with an anglaise.

Two hours before the event had started Kathy (the manager) escorted two women into the kitchen. One lady was from Iran and the other Afghanistan. They were pretty confused when I was introduced as the person running the show. They both asked, 'Who is cooking?'

'I am,' I replied.

'But you are a man?' They really were looking at something they had never seen before and it just didn't appear to be sinking in.

'When I last checked, yes, I'm a man,' I said, jokingly.

It was obviously really challenging for them to understand what they were seeing. I showed them what we were doing and what I would like them to do. One lady asked if she could taste the soup so I gave them both a spoonful for them to try. They looked like they were sort of impressed.

'It tastes ... good?' I asked, and they both nodded.

I explained that I wanted to par boil the potatoes and then drain them, toss them in olive oil and chopped garlic. I told them there was some rosemary bushes outside and they could toss some of that onto the tray.

'But that's how we would cook them!'

'Great! Then you know what I mean.'

I explained the fact that I was going to wrap the chicken with bacon and asked if they had an idea of how many people of the Muslim faith would be coming.

They explained about ten, so I said I would prepare some chicken without bacon in one part of the kitchen, and do the rest with on the other side of the kitchen.

They asked: 'You would do that for us?'

The more disbelieving they were of what I did, the more I thought: what had they seen in their lives?

They spoke to each other in their language quite a bit and looked incredulous that I washed dishes. I swept and mopped floors. They did say a few times: 'But you are a man.'

At one stage I said, 'I appreciate you come from another culture, and I respect that. But men do housework and cook in Australia. If they don't, they aren't thought very highly of.'

Augustina, Peg and Victoria had come in for the event and I had gone out to have a chat with them after their main course. I cleared the table of six in one go, stacking the plates and cutlery neatly in my right hand. I came back into the kitchen and they almost screamed with shock.

'What are you doing? You're a man!'

I had to laugh, 'Yes, men clear the tables here too!'

* * *

Augustina's Jollof Rice
Oil for cooking
Beef
Pork
Chicken breast
Shrimp
Mixed veggies
Cabbage
Parsley

START WITH YOUR OWN ONION

Onion
Canned tomatoes
Tomato paste
Salt
Stock cubes
Ground coriander

Jollof Rice is served with variations in many countries of West Africa. In Liberia, pigs' feet are used with salt pork and bacon as well as with chicken. This dish may be made from scratch with fresh chicken pieces, alone, or in a combination, but it is also an excellent dish for leftover chicken, veal, turkey, tongue, ham, bacon, etc.

1kg cooked meats such as chicken, pork, shrimp, and smoked pork
¾ cup vegetable oil
2 large chopped onions
2 green peppers chopped
½ teaspoon ground ginger
1 large can of peeled tomatoes
4 tablespoons of tomato paste
2 litres of water
3 teaspoons of salt
½ teaspoon of black pepper
½ teaspoon of thyme
1 teaspoon of crushed red pepper
2 cups of white rice
5 cups of chicken stock or water

- In a large fry pan, sauté the meats with ½ a cup

- of the oil
- In a large pot, sauté the chopped onions with the rest of the oil
- Add the green peppers and the ginger (optional)
- Once onions have sweated enough, add the tomatoes.
- Simmer for 5 minutes.
- Add the tomato paste, water, salt, pepper, thyme and red pepper
- Add the cooked meat and simmer 20 minutes longer
- In a large saucepan, cook the rice in the 5 cups of stock or water until tender
- Combine the sauce of the meat with the rice.
- Correct the seasonings with salt, pepper, etc.

* * *

Basic Cornbread
¾ cup of polenta
1 cup plain flour
¼ cup sugar pinch of salt
2 teaspoons baking soda
1 cup milk
1/3 cup vegetable oil
1 large egg

- Mix the cornmeal and milk in a small bowl so the polenta can soak while preparing the rest of the ingredients
- In a large bowl, mix together the flour, baking powder and the sugar
- Mix the egg and oil together well and stir into

the cornmeal
- Add the cornmeal to the flour and stir to moisten. Don't over mix!
- Pour into prepared pan and bake for 25 minutes or until an inserted toothpick comes out clean
- Bake only until golden brown. This recipe bakes one loaf or 16 squares.

* * *

There are some people you meet in life that I love to think are going to stay around forever. Joanne Norbury is one of those people for me. I met her at trade school where we would sit in the cafeteria and check out the male apprentice butchers, cooks, waiters and other tradesmen. After many funny and outrageous battles in the cafeteria, we came to the conclusion we have very different taste in men. We both stood out in a way because we both worked in good restaurants, whereas the majority of the apprentices worked in hospitals or old people's homes.

Joanne is – by far – a superior chef to me in so many ways. Her memory is for one, and her ability to understand the mechanics of finances. Unless I've done something many times and I haven't written it down, generally it's gone and ... well, finances were never my forte. Joanne sometimes stayed at Mum and Dad's with me when we started the year venturing into school together. The first time I showed Joanne into the bedroom, which only had a large double bed, Mum said, 'But that's your bedroom. You're staying in there, Joanne can't sleep in there!'

It was late, we had been out and we were both tired, needing to get up early to get to school. I had come out to them a few years prior to this event. Mum said it was inappropriate for a man and a woman to be sleeping in the same bed. I said: 'Mum, what do you think is going to happen?'

With that, I heard a huge burst of laughter coming from the room, which was from Joanne. Yes, I agree in so-called "normal" protocols; in those days it wasn't the done-thing, but when it involved a gay man and a woman sharing a bed, Mum had to concede that this was an area of etiquette that she hadn't thought about. Anyway, I wasn't going to sleep on the floor!

Joanne came down and worked at Queenscliff for a while. We worked really well together. We also shared the flat on Punt Road for a time. One of my favourite memories was coming home from work when Jo had the day off. I had a container of little Lindt chocolates – a hundred or so individually wrapped sweets on the table. I walked through the door to discover Jo on the couch with a stack of videos and a huge pile of wrappers from the container. She left me about three. I was shocked and laughing, calling her a greedy bitch and she just looked at me and said, sheepishly, 'I've eaten too much! I don't feel well.' It still makes me smile remembering that.

Joanne opened a restaurant on Hamilton Island where I worked with her again. An amazingly beautiful part of the world, but unfortunately the people she went into business with weren't that amazing, as I've said.

On one occasion, Joanne basically saved the skin on my arm. An apprentice had made a few breakfasts and cooked the bacon in the same pan, then placed the pan on the shelf above the gas jets where the clean pans were supposed to be kept. They were put here so during service you could easily reach and get them down to cook. It was stressed by us not to put dirty pans up there.

I came in about 10am and started to prepare for lunch

and by 11.30am lunch service had started. It got busy very quickly. I was doing the pans and got an order for risotto and grabbed the larger pan. Unbeknownst to me, the pan I grabbed had about a centimetre of bacon fat in it. As I grabbed the hot fat poured all down my arm into my arm pit and down my side.

I managed to get my jacket off as it just started to stick to the skin. Joanne was basically the only person that knew I was HIV positive on the island and so, with an emergency like this, she was invaluable. The owners wife was an ex nurse and she wanted to put hot compresses on the area. I think I was scared shitless she was going to do that. Joanne took control, got me back to my unit and carefully treated the area with cool, wet cloths for hours. I know that I would have serious scars without Joanne Norbury's quick action and amazing assistance during this time.

I remember, during our tade school years, sitting on the train going from Melbourne to Geelong and talking to an old lady when the conversation got onto making jam. I was sitting on the train talking to this older lady and over the large seat popped Joanne saying, 'I bloody thought that was your voice!' We laughed at the chance meeting. I still use the older lady's method of making jam to this day.

* * *

Making Jam

- Prepare fruit you have, discarding any brushed bits, leaves, pips, cores etc.
- If it's strawberries, take the tops off. If it's peaches or stone fruit, clean and chop, setting aside a couple of kernels for addition later

- Once fruit is cleaned and prepared, add an equal amount of sugar. This works okay, but I have learnt to add less sugar
- Say for every 500gm of fruit, add 400 gm of sugar
- Combine fruit and sugar and cover, letting it stand overnight
- The next day, strain the juice and reduce it by at least half
- Add fruit and cook till it passes the jam test (on a cold plate, put a teaspoon of jam on – if it stays in the same place and doesn't run everywhere, your jam is done)
- Towards the end, add some lemon juice to taste for a bit of zing
- You can also use a candy thermometer to judge. This method works very well for me and I use it most times making impromptu jam
- I've even made jam from left over fruit from large fruit platters. Mixed melon, grape, pineapple, apple, thrown in together and with enough sugar and some lemon zest.

* * *

Some mutual friends of Joanne and mine had a restaurant and their chef had done a runner. Jo suggested my name to them and they rang and asked me if I would do it so I took the opportunity to help out. I returned to Queenscliff where the restaurant was, and also caught up with old friends and acquaintances which was a great time – and possibly the highest paid job I had ever had in hospitality. I heard a bit later that from the time I arrived the food costs went down dramatically and there was uncertainty as to why this was so. The previous chef had left me with two freezer-loads full to the brim of food. So much so that I only had to buy fresh fruit and vegetables.

* * *

Melon and Orange Jam

This jam recipe was inspired by something Joanne showed me.

1kg melon
400gm sugar
Juices of 3 oranges and 2 Lemons
Orange blossom water, approximately 1 tablespoon

- Chop up fruit into small cubes
- Let stand with sugar, preferably overnight in the fridge, but at least for a few hours
- Drain liquid into a pot and reduce when halved, add fruit and lemon juice
- Cook till jam consistency (when a teaspoon is put on a cold plate it doesn't run)
- Just before finishing, add orange blossom water. Add half first and check the balance of flavour – if it's not strong enough add the rest
- Put into jars and seal.

* * *

Orange Marmalade

6 large oranges

GREGORY KELLY

4 lemons
8 cups of sugar
¾ cup of Scotch or orange spirit

- Cut skins away from fruit, placing flesh in one bowl and the skins in a pot of water
- Bring skin to boil and replace water 3 times
- On the third time, simmer peel partly covered until very soft and liquid equals about 2 cups
- This will take about an hour. When done, let it cool
- Chop pulp of the oranges and lemons
- Add 2 cups of cold water to pulp
- Let this stand overnight
- Cut skins into fine strips
- Strain all the pulp, discard the membrane and pips
- Now add liquid from peel
- Add the peel that has been cut into strips
- Bring to boil for 10 minutes
- Gradually stir in sugar and boil till it passes the jelly test (plop a ½ teaspoon on a cold plate, it shouldn't be runny)
- Remove from heat and stir in 3 tablespoons of scotch or liqueur
- Bottle up the marmalade and store in a cool dark cupboard
- The oranges can be substituted for blood oranges or tangelos or a combination of citrus is great.

* * *

START WITH YOUR OWN ONION

Shane Duniam, who has been such a close friend for over 25 years, and his partner Neil had moved to Central Australia and were working in an Aboriginal community. Neil was employed by the community and Shane took the opportunity to re-establish the art space. They invited me to travel up north and stay with them for a few weeks. I had to be granted special permission to stay, and felt very privileged to receive it.

This was to be a 40th birthday present from Shane and Neil to me. It really was one of the most incredible journeys I will ever take. I took the 19 hour train journey on the Ghan to Alice Springs.

The boys picked me up with new gang members, Dot and Spot – two cattle dogs they had adopted from community.

The drive out to Mimili was about five hours from Alice. We got there and I was shown around town briefly. We went back to the house, prepared a meal and ate. The next day I realised I felt challenged about walking from Shane and Neil's to the office, community store or Arts Centre. When I ventured up the street I took a wrong turn and ended up in the backstreets. It felt pretty scary – and for the first time I felt I was introduced to the real Australia.

The physical condition of some of the people, the poverty, the rubbish, the looks from some of the locals and the state of the houses were a lot to take in.

I eventually found my way to the Arts Centre where Shane introduced me to the women who were painting. I then helped out by sweeping and wiping surfaces.

A few days later, I was asked to assist in a BBQ for a special guest and several hundred other people. The HACC (Health and Community Care) building was a pivotal utility in the community. This was used daily to cook and serve about a hundred Meals on Wheels to be delivered to community members. It was a small stainless steel room with cool room walls – similar in size to a petit caravan – that had an oven, sink and a small bench. Attached to this little space was a caged veranda area where a few of us were preparing salads and such.

We were being watched by a cow called 'Moo' and a smaller bull, within millimetres of the other side of the cage, staring and dribbling at us. The bull moved away, and a camel joined Moo the cow, to dribble and stare. They were intent on me, as I was chopping about eight cabbages for the coleslaw.

I'd prepared food in some pretty interesting places, but having an audience of four legged creatures took the prize for the most interesting.

Kay, who spoke several languages, was the lady who ran the Meals on Wheels service for the community. This small area was impressively clean considering the situation. There was dust, flies, dogs and other four legged creatures, as well as the little children running around in what seemed to be a bit of calm chaos!

Neil came towards the cage with the Federal Minister of Health, Tony Abbott, along with photographers and PR people. As Tony came up to the animals, the camel moved away, but Moo remained. Tony patted the cow for a photo opportunity.

He then came into the cage where Karen (Kay's boss), Kay and I were doing the chopping. I was peeling garlic and Tony and the PR woman were saying that there had been training in the community for 20 years. I had to blurt out, 'So where is it? Where is this training?' They both looked at me, and I said, 'Oh, sorry, I'm only the ring in here!'

Tony offered to shake my hand and said, 'Hi. I'm Tony.'

'Mate, I know who you are and I just saw what you did with that cow. I'm preparing food for you to eat and I ain't touching your hand.' There was no wash basin or running water in the cage.

He put his hand away and said, 'Oh, right.'

Tony was introduced to the women and asked Karen if there was a set menu plan. She looked at him and said, 'No ...'

I felt a need to say, 'When you only have fortnightly deliveries, it's hard to rely on the chance that you will get everything you have ordered. That makes it very difficult to keep to a specific set menu. It only takes a few items not to come, and your plan is stuffed. I've been told that it can be a semi-common experience for fresh fruit to be put in the freezer section of delivery trucks and vice versa.'

'How many calories would each meal have?' was Tony's next question.

He was asking Kay and Kay nervously looked at me, so I said, 'I'm not sure how many laboratories you flew over to get here but I don't think you perceive the situation. These people are getting nourishment and a full belly, it's their only meal of the day for most of them. Asking about calories is a bit ... well ... dumb.'

He looked at the tiny kitchen and left with his entourage. I believe this was a first class example of white man discrimination in this country that I feel privileged to call home. To me, Mr Abbott seemed unprepared for the interaction of how a community worked. He never bought a painting. If he had it would have appreciated incredibly by now as, of the painters there at the time, some are in the National Gallery of Australia and it is considered an important area for Aboriginal Cultural images. A piece of the credit must go to Shane for his drive and determination in getting a small area so well established on the art world map.

The car was loaded up and food transported to the Arts Centre where the BBQ's had been set up with long trestle tables. Meat was thrown on the BBQ's and we were serving probably 200 Anangu people and Tony's entourage of about 40-odd people. Dogs ran through the BBQ's, there were flies like I'd never experienced before and there were smiles from the people.

The BBQ went very well. The elders lined up after Tony, followed by all the other adults.

The school principal, who had heard me, speaking to Tony, said, 'Well done! That was really good!'

I asked where the tji tji's (children) are. We needed the kids as there was a heap of food still to be eaten. The tji tji's came in three waves from the school.

I managed to put heaps of salad on their plates. One little guy said, 'What's your name?'

'Greg,' I answered.

'Greg, can I have some more cucumber please? I really like cucumber.' He came back three times for more cucumber.

A few kids looked as if they had to steal the fruit. One young girl slipped an orange into one pocket and a banana into the other. I think she thought I didn't see her. I picked up an apple and said, 'You need this too!'

She looked at me sort of guilty, but excited. 'Can I have that?'

'You can have as much as you like.'

This has to be one of the top three of my culinary highlights – a federal health minister and 200 Anganu people in the dirt, with several hundred dogs with all sorts of maladies, flies by the millions and children everywhere.

Tony walked past and said, 'Great coleslaw. Good tucker. Now where's this kangaroo?'

The elders had prepared a roo tail in honour of the special guest. He needed some tips on how to approach the roo tail which is a story best told by Shane. If you are offered the roo tail it is an honoured position you are being held in as generally that is for the children and elderly.

* * *

Fresh Mint Chutney

This is great with just about anything as an addition to a soup or stew or a sauce that needs oomph, two teaspoons in a dressing or as an instant marinade for cooked meat or salad.

1 cup mint
6 spring onions
1 fresh green chilli
1 clove garlic
½ teaspoon ginger
Salt
2 teaspoon sugar
1 teaspoon garam marsala
40ml lime juice

- Blitz together
- This will keep for several weeks in the fridge
- Pour a splash of oil on top to give it an airtight seal.

* * *

Candied Peel

6 oranges
2 teaspoons of bi carb of soda
1 cup boiling water
3 cups sugar
2 cups water

- Cut peel with the pith from fruit, discard stem and blossom ends
- Put in a bowl, add boiling water and bi carb
- Let stand for 2 hours
- Drain and discard the water
- Cover with fresh water and simmer till tender, which can take a while
- This water process can be repeated 3 times as this helps remove bitterness and cooked till peel is tender
- Drain, set aside
- Add 2 cups water and 2 cups sugar into a pot and bring to boil
- Pour over peel or add the peel to the pot and fold through
- Let it stand for two days
- Strain the peel from the liquid and bring liquid to boil add final cup of sugar
- Add peel and cook till peel is transparent
- Dry on a cake rack on a low heat in oven for about 20 mins
- Reduce syrup for about 20 mins and dip peel into it
- Drain and dry as before for a day or so
- And roll in caster sugar when dry
- Leave to dry before putting into container.

ELEVEN
RELATIONSHIPS AND DEATH

Cheltenham Place was a house for PLWHA's (people living with HIV/AIDS) in Adelaide set up by several support agencies. Assistance came to them by one of the nuns, Sr. Margaret, who was connected to – and helped set up – St Francis House in Melbourne. Its focus was more on respite rather than long term accommodation. I found out about the service when I was still in the country. It was about a 2 ½ hour drive one way to Adelaide to get my medication and to see doctors. For a nominal fee you could get dinner and a bed for a couple of nights to attend doctors' appointments and get medication. This is where I met Grant, Phillip and Michael – and through Grant several months later I met Merri.

Grant lived in the Clare Valley with his wife, who he later divorced. We formed a relationship of sorts over the next nine years. He is an incredibly skilled artisan – anything to do with his hands. I had not met anyone with his skill set before. In many respects I was in awe of such talent.

His house is a thick stone walled building built in the

1840's. The shed attached to the house was an old blacksmith shop where, according to local legend, the stump jump plough was invented. There is another place (I can't remember where) that also lays claim to this title. It is in this shed where he spends many hours building incredible bespoke furniture for people in the know.

Grant asked me to be an extra pair of hands while he was making a curved pelmet for a grand old house in the area. This first project together germinated an idea about my collection of dead people's furniture. An accumulation of things that had come into my life after so many funerals. Over the next five or six years he helped me transform these things into pieces of beautiful furniture that I had restored or made from scratch.

I realised that to spend quality time with him I had to be on his turf. He disliked being too social (which is a sort of contradiction considering the energy he put into catering, I know!) so we needed to have projects. I looked at what I referred to as my collection of dead people's furniture. I had my possessions that were in storage delivered and, combined with op shop bargains and Merri's generosity, I realised I had many projects that I could start. The first project was a lovely marble topped wash stand from around the 1890's that was covered in many layers of paint. Stripping the beautiful turned legs and frame of the base with caustic soda wasn't something I'd experienced before. It had intricate carved bits that needed special attention with sharp, pointy tools. Grant knew that I didn't enjoy this as I complained throughout the entire process.

Sanding was the next step. No matter that I had sanded my fingerprints off, and felt as if they'd been cauterised through the paint removal process, there was always more sanding to do! Getting the perfect finish was paramount. 'If it's worth doing, you do it well,' was Grant's motto.

I was a bit of a recalcitrant student. 'Why isn't there a machine to do this?' said I. The stripping, sanding and the layering of the French polish – each step was vital for a smooth finish. It took until I finished before I realised that each step in the process, and the attention that I needed to give to the project, were vital to the end result. In cooking, most faux pas can be covered up with sauce – not so with woodwork! Do it properly, as Grant would say, or end up with an ugly piece of furniture. The French polishing process can be quite meditative, as it needs to be applied in one smooth go. Between each polish, when it has dried, each layer is lightly sanded. After about 25 layers, it *may* be done!

I understood the effort when the job was done. When I brought the finished piece home and admired my work, I saw the end result of being a bit slack here and there. I became more aware of the passion for these jobs that Grant has. I wasn't prepared for the energy that I needed to put in, but I really loved the idea of making or restoring my furniture. My collection of other people's stuff slowly developed into my things. No matter how much I complained about the process, I loved being able to say to myself, 'Well done!'

A 1930's kitchen cupboard became the next project. Originally given to me by Michael (The Brigadier) that Dad and I had painted several years before. When Dad saw the end result, his wonderful words were spoken in true astonishment: 'Good Lord, it was such a piece of shit! It's ... it's ... magnificent!'

This is something I am really proud of. We reshaped the top levels to create one central cupboard door. In the door frame, I was able to place a wonderful leadlight window Robyn (of Thora and Robyn) made for me. It was to go into the dining room door of Two Bridges restaurant at the Winsome Hotel in Lismore. It was never installed, as Robyn completed it not long before I finished there. So it takes pride of place on the list of things I have restored or built. The list includes:

1. Building my four poster bed with gold leafed finials and, shaped into the bedhead, cut gum leaves
2. Restoring another smaller kitchen cupboard
3. Restoring seven 1930's dining chairs, originally found on the side of a road
4. Lots of miscellaneous jobs like shelving
5. Restoring a velvet covered nursing chair
6. Combining an old wooden framed mirror with a chest of drawers.

These would never have happened without Grant.

I have a collection of things I have made. When I go to God, I bequeath these to my nieces and nephews. They can sort out who wants what. I will leave it up to them. I may not have riches to hand down, but I can offer some things I've done. Along with the furniture, I have an old picture of Mum and Dad's wedding and an old photograph of a two year old Dad. Both were in damaged frames that Grant restored. These may have not survived another 50 years into the future, but with his attention there's no reason they won't last another 100. Grant gave me a photo realistic drawing of me called *God Bless the Brigadiers Houseboy* and an Andy Warhol-type painting of Mum and Dad which I love. For my 50th Grant gave me the drawing of my eyes. The painting of Mum and Dad was from a photo

START WITH YOUR OWN ONION

taken at Mum's 50th birthday party. The night when some of the guests actually had what was called in those days "full blown AIDS".

Grant became part of the Kelly family, was always included in the family gatherings, and was always asked after by Mum and Dad during our regular phone chats. Together, we did a lot of things he had never done before; from getting on public transport to travelling interstate. It would never occur to him to use public transport, which to me was odd, but he had never been to Sydney either. That seemed odder! On a trip to Sydney, we did get on public transport because driving there is just too mad.

Grant is not an emotional person. He seems to over compensate with respect to his skill base. Almost anything artistic that could be done with hands, he could do. His talents include working with precious metals, photo realism drawing, oil painting, lead light and stained glass, French polishing, furniture building and restoring, making jewellery – the list goes on and on. He is well known within his community for the jobs that no one else wants to do because they are too hard or costly. He has restored beautiful gilded old picture frames worthy of a Caravaggio, as well as restoration of the paintings themselves, and old world calendars and prints. If it could be done, he probably would know how to do it.

He is a good cook. In his environment, he likes to prepare dinner with all the trimmings. He has often said he was born in the wrong century, as he loves to bring out all his silverware. Soups in tureens, vegetables and meats are put onto different silver trays along with all the accompaniments (roast pork just can't be served without apple sauce, which is so not me!). Glasses of every different shape and size for different liquids can be a bit confusing especially after a few drinks. He took catering and hosting events at his house to the next level one year when he commissioned Merri to make a huge mosquito net for the outdoor area. It was big enough for at least twelve people and certainly worthy of a magnificent celebration. I thought I was over the top at times, but Grant certainly is far superior to me in that respect. I may think *Oh that will look good there*, but not have the skills to actually do the job, whereas Grant would know what you'd need to do to achieve the goal.

* * *

Phillip and Michael were also staying at Cheltenham Place, recovering from several health conditions. I have never seen, before or since their deaths, such dedication to the task of being a carer/partner as Phillip was. He channelled all the strength he had devoting nearly eight years of his life to Michael. Phillip's reverence to and love for Michael was so selfless in those amazing years. Being privy to some of their life's stories, I know they came together at an essential time in both their lives. Both were pretty much shattered human beings from their own life experiences. Watching them grow as a loving couple was a highlight of my life.

At first, Michael was pretty much non-verbal and Phillip did the talking – loudly! Phillip had similar characteristics to an old ward nurse that never took any shit from anyone. That nurse who implicitly knew her stuff and was not going to be told any different. We met up on a few of my trips to Adelaide before I moved to the city permanently.

I was aware that Michael had a strong connection to motorcycles. He'd had his licence taken away for a few years by the time I had met them. He could tell what sort of bike was on the road just from the sound it made. Wherever we were he'd say, 'That's a (whatever sort of) bike coming,' and he was always right.

During one conversation with Michael, it came up that I had lived in Northern Rivers. His head lifted. He smiled and said, 'Northern Rivers? Do you know Paul B?'

Surprised, I smiled and said, 'Sure do, honey! Paul B would rock up to my place on Boris (his BMW bike) with a bottle of Moet or Vodka and a bag of goodies and ask if he could stay the night! How could I resist?'

For the first time I saw Michael smile. A big broad smile. He said: 'That's Pauly!'

We spoke of people at length; of so many friends we had in common. It really was astounding that we hadn't crossed paths in the Northern Rivers. I looked away from Michael during this conversation, to Phillip and Grant. Phillip had tears in his eyes. I asked what was wrong and he said, 'You've learnt more about Michael's past in the last half an hour than I have got to know in the last six months.'

Michael's health improved enormously with Phillip's attention. His focus on detail forced doctors to complete an overhaul of all of Michael's medical conditions which were extremely complex and across state borders. This just added another layer of bureaucracy that consumed time, energy and resources. These were the absolute complex things that brought Phillip's attention to focus. Complicated levels of bureaucracy that took up time, fine-tuned his attention and gave him a purpose. If the focus was on himself, he probably would have bailed at the first hurdle, but because it was Michael he would do the obligatory cross every "t" and dot every "i". I was very humbled to be a small part of Michael's care as well as being a friend, but I was definitely more of an observer of their unconditional, male, intimate love for each other.

* * *

I rang Paul and told him of this serendipitous connection. He filled me in on his side of the story. I was aware that Paul had been a carer for several years for a close friend. I was surprised to learn that it was Michael he had been looking after. 'Gay-world is so incestuous,' as Mum would say!

The brother who took over Michael's estate when he was diagnosed with dementia sold all of Michael's assets and took over his finances.

Paul became a carer for Michael for several years. When Paul's mother was diagnosed with a serious illness, he had to give up the full time 24/7 care of Michael. He went back into the care of the family.

Paul was not given any money to assist in the care of Michael and was treated with suspicion and almost accusatory disdain by the "Christian" brother. The brother who just happened to have the control of Michael's estate. Within a few weeks of being back with the family, Michael was put into an institution in Sydney where he was raped, drugged, robbed and assaulted on many occasions. After 18 months in "The Fridge", as Michael called it, he came to Adelaide and landed at Cheltenham Place.

During his time in the institution Michael was put on the disability pension. The institution was a public (not a private) centre – which the tax payer paid for.

Phillip's attention to detail and dogged determination was put to good use when Michael had to have weekly freezing sessions on genital warts around his anus and backside. This had to happen over several months. At the end of most sessions they would come to my place. Michael not really wanting to sit, and possibly not really sure why due to

START WITH YOUR OWN ONION

his dementia. Phillip, wired on coffee, would be angry that these procedures had stemmed from his incarceration in "The Fridge". My job for those moments was to get them something to eat, some coffee, and try to calm Phillip down. If it happened to be a full moon, then Phillip was certainly on overdrive (his anti-psychotic medications sent him a bit high around full moons.)

As had happened to Paul, was repeated when Phillip took over the care of Michael. They lived in a cramped one bedroom housing trust apartment. After about three years they moved to a slightly bigger two bedroom apartment. At no stage did the brother let on to Phillip that there was a significant amount of money that could have improved their life no end. Michael received a bill for over $80,000 from Centrelink when they had moved to the two bedroom place in Magill. Phillip rang me screaming about what to do. I said you're going to have to ring the family, which he did, and to his surprise the brother said: 'Oh just send it to me, I'll fix it up.'

Michael lost the pension and his healthcare card when it was discovered that there was money to look after him. The brother then had to organise some sort of arrangement where Michael was paid a wage. According to Phillip, this distressed the brother. He had to pay Michael a minimum wage as well as full price for medications.

Michael passed away in 2010 of lung cancer. The moment he took his last breath, Phillip turned to Michael's two brothers who were there and said, 'What's the story about going to America?'

Throughout the 8 years of their relationship, Michael was very anti-American and Phillip never knew why. The brother who had the control had, many years before, put Michael and their 78 year old mother on a plane to go to some Baptist faith healing ceremony. When they arrived at JFK airport they were met with armed guards who escorted them into a small room where they were held captive for over 24 hours and then put on a plane back to Australia. The brother "didn't realise" that it was illegal for HIV positive people to go to America. He thought it was appropriate to send a man with HIV-associated dementia on a long flight with a 78 year old woman to chaperone him, but not appropriate to check the criteria for entering the country on which land he thought Michael would be healed.

This healing, I'm convinced, would've involved a quick death I'm sure. Over the 20 years that I have heard firsthand accounts of his brother's behaviour, I believe there would not have been a wish for Michael to get better. He would've had to have given the money back to Michael if he was "fully healed".

Phillip thought he would be looked after by the family after Michael's death, but ended up having to sue for any compensation. Phillip had spent a small inheritance from his mother on legal fees (approximately $20,000) and suffered huge emotional dramas, starting with the brother not wanting to give Phillip a cent. It was finally settled that the estate bought a unit for Phillip to live in for his lifetime and was given some money – absolutely nothing to compare with what he would've been given if Phillip was a female.

I was unable to go to Michael's funeral as Dad had a heart attack a few days before Michael passed away, so I was in Melbourne helping Mum.

Four and a half years after Michael passed, after a scattering of ashes on the family property about a month after his death, the brother who was in charge of Michael's estate received a phone call from the funeral directors. They asked about Michael's remaining ashes and when they would be collected. Phillip rang me to tell me of this "oversight" on the brothers' behalf. The brother had rung him and just said: 'I forgot to collect Michael's other ashes, can you go pick them up?'

The brother never explained why he had requested they be put into two containers. I was humbled when Phillip asked me to help scatter the remains in the garden bed of the house.

When I say oversight, I'm being very considerate. What I really meant to say was the brother was one of the most vile people I'd ever encountered. All under the banner of being a so called "good Christian" he basically left Michael, who was independently wealthy (we are talking millions) and had been diagnosed with dementia, to fend for himself.

* * *

Phillip passed away on the 19th of January, 2019. He had been diagnosed with bowel cancer in 2015 at the same time that Mum had been diagnosed with the same disease. Their operations were two days apart. I made sure he was stable after his operation before I headed to Melbourne to help take care of Mum.

In 2017, Phillip got the diagnosis that the cancer had metastasised to his liver. He had recently taken up horse riding again as he used to ride as a young man. He put a post on Facebook and all it said was "Bugger".

I knew he'd been to the doctors and he came straight from there to my place. I asked what "Bugger" had meant. He told me that he'd been given five years with radical chemotherapy, radiotherapy and several other procedures. The other option: two years if he did nothing. I naturally started to tear up. He looked at me and said, 'Cut that crap out. You start crying and I will not share anything with you!' He decided to go with the latter and almost made it to three years.

He was upset that he wouldn't be able to continue with riding as the drive was about an hour and a half to the ranch. I told him I'd be glad to take him and for the next two or so years I did. Sometimes he'd sleep all the way to the horses and as soon as we would get there he'd come alive.

I loved taking him up there and developed my own little rapport with Winston, Woody, Ranger and the crazy horse in the front paddock whose name I always forgot. I'd never ridden before and didn't want to venture into that area. I was happy to feed them carrots and perfect selfies with them. I was very aware this was Phillip's weekly highlight and I never wanted to encroach on his special time. His last ride was in the December of 2018, about seven weeks before he died.

Megan, the horse trainer, is a wonderful tolerant woman who trains in a way that is gentle to the horse. There's no screaming or belting the animal there is a certain psychology about her approach to horse training. She looked after between 15-20 horses that were generally discarded by others who found them too hard or difficult, or were abandoned and gave them a quality of life they never dreamed of. Winston was a favourite of mine. I posted a selfie on Facebook that was a surprise photo-bombed photo. Whilst taking the shot with him in the background, he moved his head towards mine and stuck his tongue in my ear which gave for a somewhat comical expression. After that I was in love! I got into the routine of bringing carrots and feeding them, learning things like if you drop the carrot into the dirt, don't give it to them to eat because the sand can make them sick. I thought: *Well, I wouldn't eat a carrot with dirt all over it either, but then again horses are known to eat theirs' or other horses shit!*

Phillip's knowledge on medications and procedures was extensive. He researched everything online and retained the information. For me, it generally fell out of my head. Complex words and contraindications after a few left me bamboozled. He believed he was very well equipped for the future and thought he had organised his end of life matters very well. Betty (a close friend of his for 47 years) and I were on his Advanced Care Plan. We were entrusted with speaking for him when he was unable to. I'd been through his checklist which was a folder containing all the jobs that needed to be done after he died. I didn't look that close at the time, and thought it was great until we had to deal with some of the decisions he'd made!

True to form of clashing with family events, Phillip collapsed at home in his garden the night before Mum and Dad's 60th anniversary party. Betty had left him in the afternoon as he told her to go home. He'd gone outside for a cigarette and Betty had discovered him the next morning at around 6.30am. She called the ambulance and they came and settled him in a chair. An hour or so after they had left, Betty had to call the ambulance again and later in the day a third and final time. After that, it was decided he would be put into hospital until I got back from Melbourne. He never left the hospital again and died a week later. It was very hard knowing that he had collapsed during the party and I refused to let on that anything was wrong. I didn't think it was fair to burden Mum and Dad with the news. Not on their special day.

I told him don't go anywhere whilst I was away. He laughed. I started to tell him that he couldn't die on a particular day. Gallows humour that it was, it started when he bought tickets to a concert. 'I probably won't be here so take Merri,' he said.

My reply: 'You will make the concert.'

So the joke became: 'Don't die before the Grace Jones concert, not before Alison Moyet. Not on Christmas or the same day as Aretha Franklin died.' His health had clashed with Mum and Dads serious health issues. I didn't want the conflict of being torn apart with loved ones sick in different states of the country.

* * *

Phillip's folder for death

1. **Advanced care directives:** It's worthwhile thinking about what you want when the inevitable comes along and who you want to speak for you. Do you want to be supported by machines if you are brain dead? Would you be into experimentation by medicos to extend your paralysed body? It's also vital to check every couple of years if the people that agreed to do the job – like executor, those with power of attorney, literally anyone you've entrusted your final say – still want to do it!
2. **Medical power of attorney:** It's all part of the legal process and an invaluable thing for the protection legally of the individual who has put their name on the form and will speak on your behalf when you can't.
3. **Birth certificate:** Self-explanatory, but a copy is important.

START WITH YOUR OWN ONION

4. **Tax file numbers:** Again, self-explanatory
5. **Centrelink/veteran details:** Centrelink reference numbers, any debts with information relating to them.
6. **Funeral arrangements:** Do you care about whether or not you have a funeral? How do you want your last wish on this planet to be used? Where do you want to be buried? Have you organised a plot? If you're cremated, do you want your ashes scattered? What about a natural burial in a cloth and a tree planted on you? The documents pertaining to these decisions need to be available to whomever is carrying out your wishes.
7. **Medication summary:** A list, preferably made up by your doctor, of what medications you're on. This is mainly for sudden crisis situations when your medical power of attorney and advanced care team needs to have knowledge immediately. If you have little or a lot of doctors' appointments – being able to convey any information to emergency teams is for your benefit.
8. **Medical history:** For those with a complicated history, again, it's important in an emergency to have access to any relevant information that could be useful.
9. **Will:** A copy of at least, and the relevant executor information, as well as keeping up to date as to the beneficiaries. CHANGE them if the beneficiaries die or you fall out with them.
10. **Utility accounts:** Copies of bills and

companies you deal with that will need to be closed and finalised.

11. **Bank accounts details:** Banks and institutions to contact when you die.
12. **Pin numbers to accounts:** Bank or email if relevant
13. **Possibly access to some cash:** To help if your next of kin or your advanced care people have to pay bills for you or for exorbitant parking fees and crappy food at the hospital if you think you might linger.
14. **Telephone numbers** of those who needed to be contracted at time of death.
15. **Heads of agreement:** In Phillip's case, this was the document that Phillip was forced to concede to with the brother and where he legally made Phillip give all his money to the estate of his late partner's family. All Phillip's money that he had accumulated. Life insurance, superannuation, bank balance and car. All of it Phillip was forced to give to the estate as his sign of "good faith". Settling the dispute so Phillip could have a roof over his head after eight years of love and dedicated service was not considered to be a justifiable reason to be given anything.
16. **Car registration and any insurance documents:** Papers needing to be organised with the motor vehicle office.
17. **Vehicle use:** Authorising who can use your car if you cannot. This applies to insurance and

covering your loved one's behinds if something unforeseen happens during your dying process.

18. **Distribution of possessions:** This is worthy of a conversation as to who you want to have and what you want them to have. Phillip said that he had put names on everything. Well, he hadn't, and as it was he'd left his goods to someone none of us knew. If we had taken anything after Phillip had died, technically that would be theft. Even though the brother who had already started to organise Phillip's possessions way before we had got the chance to go to the Public trustees. Again, as I conferred with the public trustee person, technically illegal. Offering a dead person's belongings to other people before you know what the will states is illegal but it wasn't an issue for this brother. Robyn had scribbled across her will that had left all her possessions to her family "NO FAMILY". She left a brief list of her things with names on it as to who she wanted to get what. This was found by Shane and Helen whilst we all were organising her possessions. A rough list written down sometime before she died and, as she had been diagnosed with an aggressive pancreatic cancer, not really enough time to get to a solicitor to make it official.

19. **Miscellaneous information:** This is all the stuff that hasn't been covered in the previous headings.

* * *

Phillip was farewelled at Rusty's Riding Retreat on the 24th of February, 2019. After I had first read his list of things to do, I brought up the fact that he had not suggested anything to do with his ashes. He told me that he didn't care.

I told him: 'Let me get one thing clear: you ain't hanging around on my mantle. I am not having a dead body in my house! I'll pick up the ashes, but you have to decide where you want to go. If you don't decide you will be put into the compost heap.' I will never forget the look of shock on his face and it still makes me smile thinking of it.

Through some Facebook posts and I believe misunderstandings on Phillips behalf (and the fact that he never spoke to his family directly on this topic), Megan suggested the ranch with the horses he loved and it was settled.

On the day of his scattering, I divided his ashes into small Chinese paper takeaway containers. I spent about 18 months collecting and drying rose petals from the rose garden at my place, these were put on top of the ashes.

We had the scattering of the ashes, I'd read my speech, and it was a sad but nice farewell with about 20 people, including Phillip's sister from New Zealand. At the end of the gathering I collected all the containers, chairs and other things I'd bought for the day, put them in my car and went home.

The next afternoon, I thought I'd better empty the car. Upon grabbing the containers I realised that there was a rattling sound as I grabbed the little boxes. Unfortunately bits of Phillip had got caught in the folds of the containers. 'Oh, Lovie,' I said to myself. 'There really is only one place for you!'

I carefully took the wire handles off the containers. All in all there were about two teaspoons of Phillip in all the containers; mainly powder, but a few "bits". I started to laugh as I put possibly his left little toe into the compost heap with the containers flattened out on top. The following days were in the mid 40's, one being 46.7C, so I'm sure he's nicely cooked through my compost.

It was a sad lonely death. No family. Betty and I who were long term friends, but only let in on some things. He was anally private and, looking back, somewhat paranoid about the circles he lived in and not mixing those circles. That is so un-me!

* * *

Merri, a close friend of Grant's, was part of the quartet. I had the pleasure to meet her in the early days of my moving to Adelaide. Not long after I moved into my apartment, her mother had to be put into care. I was asked by Grant to help move things out of her mother's home and Merri offered anything I needed.

Arriving in Quorn where Merri's mothers' house was, I made the dumb decision to drink wine. It was not my intent to drink a lot of wine, but probably a combination of a long drive, life in upheaval, getting over an infection and trying to keep up with the others, I got awfully pissed. I remember going on a tour of the pubs and the next day being so sick like I've never been before. That was the last time I ever got shamefully drunk. Sixteen years later I still get the shudders remembering how drunk I was!

I'd agreed to a deal to help clean up the house and in return anything that caught my eye was on offer. I don't recall fulfilling my end of the bargain. I managed to get back to the Clare Valley to Grant's, but it took at least a week to recover. I was given a mattress and household things including an octagonal little coffee table made by Merri's grandfather in the 1890's – all very handy to "instantly" have.

Merri has five children, and when she moved to Adelaide a year before me, she had her three girls still living at home. Her youngest daughter is Maddy and, as Merri said at the time, 'Ten years old – going on twenty-one.'

Over the years, Grant and I were invited to many BBQ's and it always felt like we were part of the family. Many BBQ's, salads, dips, cakes and glasses of bubbles have been consumed at Merri's under the verandah at the back of her house. She's an incredible reader, consuming about three books a week, and is a very deep-thinking, emotional woman. She has all my respect and admiration as a dear friend as well as a single mother who raised five children on her own. Four of the five went to university and all are achieving successful lives. They all had music in their childhoods, either singing and or learning to play instruments. Merri has been a minister, a choir master and a member of many choirs', a primary school teacher, a dance teacher as well as a music and singing teacher. She has been involved in theatre – from directing, acting and as the costume designer and costume maker. Merri has made beautiful clothes and cushions for me with stitching that would drive me insane trying to do! I have a beautiful vest of dark blue velvet and light blue ribbon and a cushion of material from a costume I wore in a play that we were in together. The stitch is called cathedral window patchwork quilting. It's incredibly intricate and I assume meditative to do, but a job I don't believe for me. She is the inspiration for me to take the random collection of stories that were badly written by me to what this is today. She painstakingly has read and corrected at least eight drafts of this book. Without her this would never have seen the light of day.

In about 2011, Merri asked me to help her get into town as she had an appointment. We had done the things she needed to do and we were walking up Rundle Mall and I was saying to Merri: 'Mum thinks the gay world is all closely connected.'

I looked across from the Balls sculpture and saw a woman who was looking at me with a look of shocked surprise on her face. I looked at her and studied her face. It took a few seconds and I said, 'Liza … ?' So, not only was gay world small, but here appeared another friend I'd not seen for at least 20 years.

'Greg! Oh my God!' she said. Here standing before me was the grown woman who I last saw as about a 21 year old. It's just wonderful to have that moment of chance recognition of serendipitous splendour! She had been living in Adelaide for a while and, as she was around the time of the War Years, she had assumed that I had gone to meet my maker. We spoke excitedly, had lots of hugs and committed to connect for dinner. Since then this has happened many times as well as wonderful surprise visits in the late afternoon with champagne and dinner.

Liza was in a powerful position within the banking industry. I was, at that first moment of reconnecting, and always will be, absolutely delighted and ecstatic that a "girl from the bush" had gone so far. I felt incredibly overwhelmed that I had caught up with her again. It is another full circle moment in my life and it's the women that always play the integral parts of my feeling complete. My Earth Mother Goddesses keep the wheels turning!

* * *

About 10 years ago I was part of a conversation over lunch

with Grant and Merri. I probably wasn't paying attention so I didn't realise who they were talking about, but a man's Christian name was mentioned. It happened to be the same name of a man that was in the housing co-op I was in. It just happened to be an unusual name. It just happened to be him! They were talking about Maddy's father who, before this time, I never thought was any of my business to ask about. I just knew him as a rather hard to get to know, aloof, gay man.

For over ten years I had kept the knowledge to myself until the night when the co-op was having its last meeting ever. As the meeting was in progress, the motion being read was to hand over the management of the houses to an association. A winning show of hands rose that didn't think highly of me for whatever reason – I don't care.

I spoke with real appreciation that I was able to be a friend of a great family and an observer of now a young woman who is very talented (and he missed out by inference). I felt I didn't belittle the situation by being nasty or telling him what I thought about his role as a father, just that he has a wonderful daughter.

* * *

Honeycomb

1 ½ cups sugar
½ cup honey
1/3 cup water
2 tablespoons of golden syrup
2 teaspoons of bi-carb soda

- Place baking paper on a tray chosen for the

honeycomb, wipe a trace of oil over the baking paper – this is best done with paper towel
- Bring the sugar, water, honey and golden syrup to 155C on a candy thermometer
- Let it stop bubbling for a minute, then add bi-carb
- Quickly stir it through it will froth quickly, be aware as to not scald yourself
- Pour onto the tray
- If you add a few teaspoons of cardomam or ground ginger (or both) to honeycomb when adding the bi-carb it adds an interesting touch.

* * *

As far as relationships go, I don't seem to have been that good at them. Most of my teen years and early adulthood were spent with thoughts of: *Why aren't I good enough? I must be so evil to have the desires I have. No one will love me. Am I that unlovable that I will burn in hell? Obviously I am ugly no one loves me.* Or being just really self-deprecating. In fact, I had a whole collection of self-doubt and negative self-image thoughts, which sometimes still rear their ugly head.

I suppose I wanted what everyone else seemed to have naturally, but the Church and the school yard told me how bad I was and that left a lasting impression. I was quite consumed with the idea of not ever being good enough to have someone to love me. Many nights I sobbed myself to sleep feeling not worthy enough, but never really knowing why. I felt that I had a void in my soul – that I was one of God's rejects. I was the odd one out, the one that was picked on. Early in my adulthood when I did come out I felt I would fulfil the prophecy, said to me by "kind", "concerned" people: 'Oh you are gay. That's sad. You will be old and lonely.'

I believed it was my choice to be gay but was not in touch with myself enough at the time to understand it was my choice to be happy with who I was and what I was given (genetically speaking). It was a choice to be true to myself, not a choice to be gay like one chooses strawberry filling over chocolate.

To this day, I haven't had a lover say they loved me (Mitchell did say it a few times, but considering his emotional and physical violence I have decided that I don't and didn't believe him). How my life may have been so different if an honourable man who I respected had said to me as a child that the negative thoughts I was thinking were not true. That I am worthy and what I was feeling about being a male attracted to men was definitely okay. Alas, it didn't happen and I spent a long time having a very negative self-image. Since my studies in mental health I have strived to become that honourable man and have spoken to the lost frightened lonely little boy that I was. I think I have resolved my issues with him, but every so often the scared little insecure boy can rear his head. Although, this time, with knowledge gained and the strong fabulous people in my life, I can choose to not let him rule my actions. I have the knowledge and belief in the people around me. I know implicitly that if I am low and sad I have to remember that I am respected and loved. I also know if I'm being a drama queen my friends will tell me to pull my head in!

Moments that take me by surprise when I am focused on other things is when people can get under my emotional armour. One of my earliest memories of school is Mum dragging me down the street to attend. I was hysterical and just didn't want to go. I think in a childlike way the name calling had already begun and I knew I didn't like it. I was five years old. Nowadays, I would say I suffered from a good dose of anxiety – then, I was called a naughty boy.

* * *

I first met Emmanuel through Elizabeth and I met Elizabeth through my volunteer work at Bay FM radio. I had the night time slot, midnight till 3am. My show was called *the Black Brahms and Boogie Show*. This gave me enough scope to play anything from soul gospel dance to classical. Elizabeth was the secretary of the station and we hit it off almost instantly. I would come in during daytime hours to help on the front desk, do filing or whatever needed doing. One such job was to sign about a hundred certificates for people that had donated a few dollars to the station. I asked if I could sign her name on these certificates for her. Her surname has p's and r's and t's – great to add flourish on a certificate. So I showed her a practice of how I would sign her name and she loved it. As I was going through the certificates, her name got more extravagant the more I did. We have a giggle about those days.

Manny and I saw a bit of each other in the early days but our relationship is now purely platonic. He is one of the few men in my life that has bridged that great divide from lover to friend. He is unique. He is a great cook, taught mainly by his mother and years of experience in kitchens. It is a mother's touch that I most admire in anyone's cooking – and he has it. Fancy, dainty food is fine in its place; however, wholesome, nourishing goodness is really what makes a person go. The ability to look at ingredients and to come up with ideas for an end result is a skill that we all need, and Manny has that. This was an important skill when he worked for me at the Winsome Hotel. My brain would be exhausted at times and it was so important to have another person whose opinion and skill I trusted implicitly, who could take up where I was dwindling.

There is a dish from Manny's family called Gux Ma Gux, pronounced "Goosh ma Goosh", which I understand to be 'A bit of this and a bit of that'. It's a curry powder and potato based dish with a large selection of different meats made into a crumble/baked stew. The list of different meats is somewhat challenging in today's world but it is a dish of its time. All food can have a time and place. There is a time for Beluga caviar just as there may be a time in everyone's life for a dish that will fill you when you are starving. This is definitely a dish that was about stretching a relatively cheap ingredient at the time – which was meat – to feed a large family. I love a family history recipe that has been given down over the generations. It's a holy grail. A recipe or meal, an essential part of life, that has nourished and kept everyone alive, enough that is to have a history itself. That a recipe has fed and been spoken of by my grandfather and will be spoken of by his great, great grandchildren is a connection that I know I am privileged to have. Whether it's Gux Ma Gux or Mum's Pavlova, I am aware that many generations have loved and love Mum's Pavlova's and that is wonderful. I am connected to so many people through her speciality. They are part of the ribbon that binds the ties.

Mum called Friday nights "Catch as Catch can" at our house. Growing up, when we were teenagers, we could have whatever was in the fridge. The condition was: we had to cook it. I know if I cooked on these nights I experimented with stews and soups that were all a bit throw it all in and see what happens. One of my older brothers, Paul, was lucky enough to have a sort of home economics class and he brought home what became a bit of a family favourite a dish called Mexican Sausages. I'm not sure what was Mexican about it, but it was another opportunity for Mum to have a break when Paul made it. It involved boiling sausages and cooking them with onions in a tomato soup. Something I've not repeated.

The statistics on food wastage in the West are phenomenal. About eight billion dollars in Australia alone I've heard. Both Manny and I hate waste – maybe this comes from our backgrounds. Over the years he has assisted me in many of my hospitality ventures and we always enjoy cooking with each other. Sometimes we have cracked the shits with each other when working in strenuous situations, but we always laughed at the end.

Many of my close friends have been – or are in – the situation of being a carer to their respective parent or parents. Manny helped care for his mother for 12 years till her passing just before her 101st birthday. I had a major life highlight by going to Malta and, after years of knowing Manny and only hearing stories of some of his brothers, sisters, nieces, nephews and great relations, I finally got to meet a whole swag of his family. The special part was meeting his mother, who generously let me stay in her house for the time of my holiday. We travelled all over Malta and Gozo, as well as a trip to Paris which included *Madam Butterfly* at the Opera Bastille and individual ballet performances all throughout the Palais Garnier. I could never repay the kindness shown to me for this extra ordinary experience.

It is I think the greatest thing that we as humans can do is to care for loved ones in their declining years. Robyn, Shane, Phillip and Manny have always inspired in me such respect for their ability to devote their life to caring for loved ones.

* * *

Nougat
2 cups sugar
1 cup water
1 cup glucose
½ cup honey
3 egg whites
Rice paper

- Line a tray 20x20cm with baking paper (light spray of oil or wipe with a paper towel)
- Or, on top of the baking paper, line up sheets of rice paper that the nougat will be placed onto
- Add sugar, honey, water and glucose into a pot and dissolve together
- Separate into two saucepans half-half
- Bring one mixture to 130C
- Whip whites in mix master and when they peak pour in 130C syrup
- Keep whipping
- Bring second mix to 156C
- Add to beating mix and beat until room temperature (a long time)
- Pour onto a tray that is lined with rice paper or baking paper
- Place rice paper on top to help push it into shape. Let it set
- It may go quite hard but will soften in a few days in an airtight container

- By adding (close to the end of process) 80gm of melted chocolate, cocoa or drinking chocolate, you can make chocolate nougat. Fold through nuts and dried fruit or chopped fine ginger and candied peel before putting onto tray.

* * *

I've had very similar themed conversations with many gay men who have gone from hetero to homo relationships. On one such occasion, admittedly, I was feeling a bit sorry for myself – a bit self-indulgent maybe – and I was complaining about not having a lover and I turned to the gent I was talking to and he replied, 'I know how you feel. It's taken me years to find one.'

I was hurt when he said that, as I was aware of his heterosexual past. I replied that he had been married 20 years and had children and grandchildren and had he disregarded them?

'I was talking about my true self,' he said.

I told him that he had stood in front of all his family, professed a love for, and was able to have love professed to him. His children had accepted his new lifestyle and that was even more fortunate.

Sometimes I wonder what makes a man. Just how far removed from his chromosomes he can go to find happiness over "fitting in". I've witnessed some men who come out later in life after being married and having children. Sometimes I find they don't seem to realise that they have dropped a live bomb on their partners' and children's laps by coming out. It can be all about them. 'Oh my children don't love me anymore because I'm gay.' Maybe it's not because you're gay but you've shattered their perception of you. They have to learn to know the person they thought they knew implicitly, all over again. These situations will take all the time they need to heal – if they ever will.

Not often, but I have occasionally been envious of men that have had a hetero marriage, children, picket fence and all that. After experiencing that to then come out and get a man. Many don't seem to be able to realise how fortunate they are. It's like shopping for ingredients: some people have never found the shelves bare.

To have one relationship male or female is a success where love was professed openly and without ridicule or scorn. I still hope for a loving relationship, but I feel possibly I will be another spinster keeping up with tradition in the line of spinsters on Dads family tree.

My experience with Mitchell scared the crap out of me. When Grant and I started seeing each other very early on it was clear we were from totally different experiences in life. He, for one, was still married and in a somewhat non-functioning situation. He could be very distant emotionally and was tactile phobic. I'd never met anyone before who hated the idea of a massage. I was very aware of the irony that I did a massage course to help my sex life and the person I meet cringes at all my best moves! In a karmic sort of way getting my fingers burnt by Mitchell, it made sense that I would attract a man like Grant into my life. Sort of once bitten twice shy.

If I put a barrier around my heart it would be safe, and for quite a few years it was – and then I had the heart attack!

* * *

Mum and I were recently talking, there was a reference to

START WITH YOUR OWN ONION

childcare centres and Mum said, "The first few years of a child's life are so special and precious. I was very grateful that I had been able to stay home and look after my children."

I totally understand that and I'm never going to have children! I also believe the last few years of life have a similar quality. Obviously, death doesn't come when we want it to, it can happen at any moment, but as some of us are fortunate to live long lives, spending time with parents in their later years I believe is an honour.

There is no point if you get to the end and some of your last words are: 'I should have said,' 'I wished I had done,' 'I should have spent more time ...' or any other statement that comes from regret.

I was sitting in a men's circle at a festival and the talking stick was going around. Many men were talking about their fathers and how bad they were. When it came time for me to speak I said, 'First off, I'm not speaking to anyone specifically, but ... I hate you all. You symbolise all the bullies that picked on me at school. I'm the only gay man in this group and I bet you guys would have given me a hard time in the playground at school. If you didn't, you didn't come and rescue me from the ones that were bullying me.' They agreed that was possibly the case. I went on to say: 'I have forgiven you. It took a long time, but I have. Your fathers may have been awful but, unfortunately, what you got was all they had to give. They didn't have the skills to sit around and talk about feelings.

'You've all said that because your fathers were bad you were scared how you were going to relate to your children. The fact is: you are talking about it, so you are okay. Your fathers did the best they could. If it was crap then think about what his life was like at a similar age and the things that he was exposed to. He didn't probably know any better.

'You are all men now, and you all need to deal with what happened in the best way you can. By talking about it here, you are. Continuing to talk about your issues is a skill that, inadvertently, your fathers gave you. You know what he didn't give you; therefore, you know what you must give your children.'

* * *

The only thing Letho was more passionate about than Mozart was his parents. He studied music extensively, but his dedication to his mother as her prime carer and his father was humbling to watch. He's a very appreciative diner and when he was living in the apartment downstairs from me I would often call him up for dinner or send a text saying 'Cafe?' It was always good to see him for his enthusiasm about my food as well as his company.

I first met him when working for the AIDS council of SA at a function and he was with the multicultural sexual health team. He has an expression on his face when he puts something in his mouth that he likes. His eyes roll, his face relaxes into a *"UUMMMM"*. A very similar look of appreciation as does Bronwyn. He honoured me by writing a piece of music for me in the style of Mozart as a birthday gift. Letho, after a few moves, ended up in Tasmania where his parents went into care and he was their primary carer. After about 11 years of being by their side, Helen passed away and, six weeks later, Letho's father Jim followed her. It takes many years to overcome the grief that can follow situations like this. My dear friend moved back to SA and has found himself a little niche in the country with a great collection of new friends and he's back doing what he loves: music.

If there is a relationship "type" that I most adore in my life it is the one where my significant other or others are eating and appreciating my food. Letho and his parents loved my olives, also my candied peel, jams, liquors, cakes and biscuits and I love an appreciative audience.

I'm really proud I have given olives to Greeks and Italians who have given me the thumbs up. I've given jam to old ladies who have asked for more. I have impressed incredibly wealthy people with my humble skills which is gratifying. It's easy to think money can buy anything, but love and passion are two things that it can't. I have worked in soup kitchens where there has been an audible silence when the eating is being done and then spontaneous laughter and merriment on completion. That truly is close to a divine experience. I've had thunderous rounds of applause for the food I and the teams I've worked with have prepared. Knowing the job is done and there has been nourishment and good vibes passed on is the thrill. A meal made with a bit of love and passion can lead to the most spontaneous conversation and healing experience.

I know when death happens – when a bereaved partner or family is in shock, when friends and family start descending into grief, sharing the tragedy – food is one of the last things on people's minds. On these occasions I have arrived with sandwiches, soup or whatever and feel that addressing a need is a way of sharing. I've seen depression set in when people can't or won't eat and it does no one any good. I know the dead person wouldn't be happy to be used as an excuse to not carry on with life.

In a very powerful counselling class during my diploma, my lecturer told me to put my leg around the leg of a chair and to drag it along as I walked. She then pointed out that the chair was all my dead friends and I was carrying them around impeding my growth. I was stuck in sadness and guilt about why I was still here and they were all dead.

One such occasion of a sudden death was the brother of a dear friend, Michelle; he had lost his life in a car accident. Michelle had a shop up the road from where I worked. She was an amazing florist and her shop was always beautiful. When I heard that this tragedy had happened, it was also said that there were people coming from everywhere to grieve. Our kitchen made trays of food and I took them up to her place. It was a way of acknowledging the tragedy with some practicality.

A couple of times a week I would pop into Michelle's shop with pieces of cake or chocolates and I would swap these for a few blown roses using the petals on desserts as garnish. One time I had made a croquembouche for a wedding and, unbeknown to me, the waiters had put it under the heating vent. There was some time before it was to be served and I happened to look out into the restaurant to see the tall, meter-high wedding cake had reshaped itself to a bowed circular shape. I grabbed the Maitre D' and pointed it out to him and it was brought into the kitchen in a panic. I ran up to Michelle, describing what had happened and she gave me several metres of beautiful ribbon. I spiralled the ribbon up the dessert, splashed it with rose petals and pulled it back into shape. Michelle saved the moment. The customers thought they had two desserts.

I had the opportunity to design a dress for my sister Libby and had it made for her birthday. I was describing it to Michelle a few days before giving the dress to Libby. The next day, Michelle rang me and asked me to come to the shop before giving Libby the dress. She had made a gorgeous headband of apricot baby roses for my big sister.

* * *

It is said that sex work is the oldest profession. I say that's bullshit. A person has to eat before they can breed. So I say cooking has to be the oldest. We have to eat before building, making tools, ploughing fields or having sex every day! Possibly the only older profession is gathering the food before eating.

I love the little hints that one gets in food-related conversation, like when Letho's father told me about olive brine: 'The brine is ready when you can float an egg on it and the diameter of a twenty cent piece of the egg is sticking out of the water.'

Ivana shared many tips on pasta. This one stayed with me: 'When rolling your pasta, it is ready when, with your hand receiving the rolled sheet of pasta, your fingertips do not make any impression on the finished sheet (from the underside).'

'Cakes, meat loafs, meat patties terrines will feel firm to the touch when they are fully cooked.'

Sue's never fail fabulous roast pork crackling method: 'Put the leg onto a cake rack over the sink and pour a jug of boiling water over the scoured skin before cooking. Then, rub a good amount of salt into the fat. Into a hot oven for half an hour then turn oven down to continue cooking.'

One such interesting hint from the *Fowler's Method of Bottling Fruits and Vegetables* (22nd revised edition), I quote: 'To peel the peaches it is usual to use caustic soda water, generally spoken of as lye.' The idea was to blanch the peaches in hot caustic soda water to help get rid of the skins. If caustic wasn't around you could use washing soda. Then, after blanching, they were refreshed in cold water where the skins would come off. My gut reaction to this hint was not to follow through on that one! The idea that caustic soda was used at any stage of cooking is bizarre.

I remember one time at Queenscliff Hotel when one of the kitchen hands tried to use caustic soda to remove burnt residue from an aluminium pot. We had to evacuate the kitchen whilst the fumes cleared.

* * *

I found "my space" within our large family in the kitchen as a young pre-teen. It was where I was validated. I got praise from Mum that I took a job away from her and generally from my brothers and sisters I got compliments. 'Oh, great! Greg is cooking.'

I was happier organising the pantry with its burgeoning shelves than I ever was on a football field. I would pull things off the shelves, wipe the shelves down and refill old Pablo and Maxwell House glass coffee jars so they were full with flours and powders for the next round of baking. I'd get on a roll and make trays of chocolate crunch and raspberry shortcake, peanut biscuits and all sorts of goodies and there was an appreciative audience.

I have learnt that with just about any savoury thing you can do, it starts with an onion. Soups, stews, casseroles and sauces – whatever one is making: sweating the chopped onion till it's clear and then adding the garlic is the best start to any dish. Even if the onion gets too much colour (not meaning burnt) it can still be rescued by adding liquid to boil the residue from the bottom of the pan. Once the onion is cooked, then the garlic added, the hard vegetables (carrots, celery leeks). Next, spices of any sort – or maybe they are sprinkled on the meat – so the meat would be next, then the liquid.

People ask me: 'How can I come into a home and make a meal when I have never been in that kitchen?'

Start with the basic questions: How many for the meal? What's in the cupboard and fridge? Are there farinaceous things like rice, pasta, potato, beans, cous-cous, flour gnocchi, or polenta? Is there meat, a can of tuna or a main ingredient meat alternative? Are there vegetables and something to make a sauce with like wine or stock? If it has an Asian theme, is there coconut milk or powder? Possibly it could have an Italian, Spanish or Mexican flavour, so is there a can of tomatoes? These questions can be answered quickly by a simple observation that will lead to a full belly for all concerned.

I suppose, just like a good relationship, a cupboard needs a certain list of ingredients that needs adding to every once in a while. Maybe that's where I have failed: I haven't kept up with the changing ingredient list.

So I've decided I can only help myself – and start with my own onion. Do the best I can and realise that I obviously needed to go through everything I have to get to where I am today. I could begrudge where I am today and say I wanted more, but I've pretty much always had enough. My cupboard of life skills overflows with some absolutely extraordinary people and experiences that have been integral to what makes me who I am today. They have all been the seasoning to my life; the thing that has made it so rich in flavour and substance.

I am very blessed to have the angels that I have. Starting with Mum, Dad, our grandparents (even the one that wasn't there), my brothers, sisters and to you nieces and nephews, and all my Earth Mother Goddesses and dear friends.

I was never that receptive when people were telling me what to do. I was told by an older apprentice many years ago when the chef came up in conversation. Everyone seemed to agree that this particular chef was an arsehole, the apprentice turned to me and said, 'Anyone can be an arsehole. The thing is, if you learn from him, that's great. When you get to a point when you aren't learning anything, then it's time to go.'

If a person has value or impact in your life and their behaviour is challenging, then the value of what you are receiving from that person is weighed up against the challenging behaviour. The time when you are constantly dealing with situations and not getting the love back (or the important information) is time to address your motivations. There's no point in trying to wait for them to change because they won't. It is all you.

* * *

If there is one thing that I would like to say to you Benjamin, Damian, Aaron, Joshua, Samuel, Lucas, Jordan, Gemma, Aidan, Finn, Tara and Jayden: never have regrets. This life is so quick, so fleeting, too much time can be spent on 'what ifs ... !'If you can deal with something on the spot then do it, but there are some circumstances you need to step back from. Life has given me many exercises in timing. If you need to make amends with someone – do it now. So many friends I saw got to the end of their life and said, 'I should have done ...'

This is a tragedy and a lesson that has been really powerful in my life. When I looked up into the sky on King

William Road, heart feeling like it was going to explode, with no one around and I realised this could be it, I had a powerful exercise in my faith in me. I didn't want to die. I had too much going on, but whatever was going to happen ... I had to let it be so. I asked all my dead friends for help and they came through. I was helped in the most powerful of ways. In the darkest hours, when the train wreck is in progress, this is when my faith was tested. Not a religious faith, but faith in me and a trust of the situations that I put myself in – they are for my best. Life is pretty damn fabulous and just who would have ever thought that I would live to see 50! Certainly not me. I know I have met and am helped by countless angels. My heavenly choir consists of joint rolling, hard drinking, wild partying, fabulously creative and joyous, sometimes conservative angels. Xx

* * *

Hot and Spicy Banana Ketchup
 1 cup raisins
 ¾ cup roughly chopped onion
 3 or 4 large cloves of garlic
 2/3 cup of tomato paste
 2 ½ cups of apple cider (or white) vinegar
 2 kilos of really ripe if not blackening bananas
 4 to 6 cups of water
 1 cup brown sugar
 1 teaspoon cayenne
 4 teaspoons of allspice
 1 ½ teaspoons grated nutmeg
 1 teaspoon ground pepper
 ½ teaspoon ground cloves
 1/3 cup of dark rum (brandy or scotch tequila)

- Put raisins, onions, garlic and tomato paste into a blender to make a paste.
- Add some of the vinegar if needed
- Scrape puree into pot and heat to give this mix a bit of cooking (beware the vinegar can 'clean your lungs' a bit)
- Puree bananas and add them to the pot, then add the rest of the vinegar, 4 cups of water, brown sugar, salt and cayenne pepper
- Bring mixture to boil and then turn down on a low heat
- Add rest of ingredients (except booze) and cook for about an hour
- If it looks like it is starting to catch on the pan (stick or slightly burn) then add more water
- It needs to cook long enough that it thickly covers the back of a spoon (or when you drop a teaspoon on a cold plate it doesn't run everywhere)
- If you like a really fine sauce this can be put back into the blender
- When you think its cooked enough add the spirit and stir bring to a quick boil
- Test for tart, sweet, salt, fruit acid by tasting adjust to your liking and then bottle
- Leave it for at least a few weeks before using. It should last for about a year in the cupboard. Once opened, keep in the fridge.

***

Mum's Relish

6lb (nearly 3 kg) of tomatoes

START WITH YOUR OWN ONION

2lb of onions
2lb of sugar (brown, raw or white)
½ teaspoon cayenne pepper
6 tablespoons plain flour
3 tablespoons of mustard powder
2 tablespoons curry powder
2 x ½ cups of salt

- Blanche and skin the tomatoes
- Chop onions
- Cut tomatoes into quarters
- Place into a dish and sprinkle with ½ cup salt
- Into another bowl, place chopped onions sprinkle with the other ½ cup of salt
- Cover both trays and let stand overnight
- Drain the residue from both bowls
- Put tomatoes and onions into a pot and boil for 5 minutes with the vinegar
- Add the sugar, cayenne and mustard boil this for about an hour
- Mix the plain flour and curry powder into a paste and add to the mixture and boil for a further 5 minutes
- Bottle whilst hot.

* * *

Shane's Mango Sauce

2 mangoes
A little chilli
A splash of fish sauce
2 cloves chopped garlic
A small knob of chopped or grated ginger

A good squeeze of lime juice
A small bunch of chopped coriander
A splash of cider vinegar

- Put ingredients all together. Mangoes can be chopped or pureed. All the ingredients can be pureed together or chopped chunky or fine as you can.

The above sauces are fabulous and can be served with almost anything seafood, red meat, vegies and poultry. This is great at a BBQ or for a formal dining meal, great as a gift and relatively cheap to make.

*** * * ***

My diary notes about Robyn (Robbie)
Lismore NSW
September 11 2015

My dear friend is dying and my heart is breaking. She is in severe pain that is trying to be wiped out by heavy duty drugs but more what they are really doing is creating a mental confusion within Robbie.

We had dinner tonight Shane, Neil, Robyn and myself. I had made cannelloni. There was some issues that hadn't been organised yet a small legal issue, car repairs and there had been a phone call from a girlfriend of Robyn's who had only spoken to Neil and not Robyn. She wasn't happy about that at all. I think she is feeling a loss of control and she got upset.

We rallied and got her focused on that she had put on weight up to 40.9 kilos. When she rang me to tell me of her diagnosis she was 37 kilos. After dinner we sat on the verandah and had a smoke after which she decided to go to bed.

Thora, her mother had always asked me, no matter the weather, if I was wearing a singlet. It became a bit of a catch phrase.

As I escorted her to bed Robyn said, 'Have you got a singlet on?'

My reply, 'Darling with all the angels around you I wouldn't dare not have one on!'

We both laughed and then she grabbed me tighter and sobbed into my arms.

September 19 2015

I've been here for 11 days and Robyn's deterioration has been rapid. The other day we were in the kitchen together and she was standing next to the wall calendar. She asked me, 'Now when are you going away?'

I'd planned a trip away a 50th birthday present to myself; my first overseas trip in 30 years. It had been booked for months.

I said to her, 'I've booked to leave on the 25th so the latest is probably the 23rd I would have to get back to Adelaide to pack but I'm thinking I should postpone it.'

She looked me in the eye and said, 'You're getting on that plane! I won't be here when you get back. I will not have it. You must get on that plane and have a fabulous time. I demand it!'

That was some of the last coherent words I had with her. Talking and ability to focus on this earthly level has left. Her attention has turned to dealing with her imminent death.

I want to use the word strong but it's not really accurate.

I'm being in control of my personal emotions. I know Robbie doesn't want a blubbering old thing like me at her side.

We sit with her and wait. She hasn't eaten anything for about a week. In a vain sort of way it occurred to me that I had prepared the last thing she ate, until a nurse during a quick trip to hospital gave her some chocolate pudding.

I am torn in half. In a week from today I'll be in Malta and more than likely Robbie will be gone. Moments of just pure anguish overwhelm me and I take some time out for a walk in the garden to weep.

We found out at the hospital that the weight she had put on was in fact the tumour had doubled in size.

Shane, Neil, Helen or I didn't get much sleep in the last week or so. We gave her the best environment for her passing we possibly could. All her needs we tried to meet.

Watching her in so much pain was excruciating. She was hospitalised to get the pain under control and when she was released Neil had driven her back home. The front entrance has about 20 steps and the house is on stilts above the 1 in 100 year flood level. I opened the car door for her and asked if I could carry her up the stairs. I got a stern look and an emphatic, 'No.'

Shane and I held her as she was determined to get up the stairs. Never have I seen such a brave and heroic (stubborn) thing. It took quite a while to get her up as she kept standing on her socks, but she got there. We got her into bed and she slept.

We had all thought she was going to pass on the Sunday night but in the morning she still had very laboured breathing clinging to life. That evening after a meal we went in and sat by her bed. I lay on the bed next to her until about 12.30. I stroked her hair as we all told funny stories about Robbie to each other.

I went to bed about 1am and left Helen with Robbie. About 3am I woke to hear her breathing had changed it was louder and almost orgasmic continuous moaning. I got up again and went in to be with her.

We said to her that her time has come, She was free to go. We love you so much. Go to your Mum. Thora is waiting for you.

Robbie at one stage said a very soft 'Mummy.'

September 22nd 2015

It has happened, my dear Robyn passed away at 4.15am on the 22nd of September. I will always thank the God's above that I was able to be with my dear friend at this time.

I went and woke Shane and Neil. We cried and played music Fly Robin Fly x

Shane and Helen attended to her body with a lavender bath and oil. She was laid with her hands crossed over her chest and flowers from the garden were picked and placed on and around covering her.

September 25th 2015

Emirates flight Adelaide to Malta. No time to grieve. Life goes on and I'd been commanded to enjoy myself. I can't describe how I felt other than privileged to be able to be with Robyn, to be on this trip and to be alive.

APPENDIX

Adelaide has been very good for my public speaking abilities I was asked to participate for a few years running in candlelight vigil ceremonies which I still consider to be a great honour. I've been asked to write articles in different magazines and here is a collection of some of those.

World AIDS Day Speech

What is important to me?

The important things are my parent's family and friends and not just in a crisis but always and personally challenging myself to be inspired, to experience as much as possible and to live without regret.

What keeps me going?

I am kept going by a healthy expression of who God made me to be knowing that "one day he'll come along" and by acceptance of my journey fundamentally knowing that this game we play called life has purpose meaning and is fulfilling.

APPENDIX

What inspires me?

I am inspired by better medications, and that I was born in Australia and not any other country because I am aware that I am a recipient of the best public health services in the world.

Gregory Kelly 1/12/08

* * *

Phillip's Ashes Ceremony

Welcome

I would like to start by acknowledging the traditional owners of this land and pay respect to elders past and present.
    I would also like to acknowledge Megan and Steve and I can't thank you enough for your visits to Phillip in hospital and for letting him be here in the end.

We are here to honour our family member and friend with his last wish ever.
    This is not a time for good byes just good memories and please remember this is not a funeral. Phillip made his wishes very clear that he did not want one of those and threatened a haunting if he got one! He threatened to haunt me if I did other things I said Great I'll take pics! But in saying that I'm sure he would be very surprised as to the turn out today. Thank you everyone for being here.

What Phillip had no time for was that gatherings like this

APPENDIX

don't have much to do about the person who has gone but its about us who are left behind. Us who are reminded that we also wait for our own turn. Us who have gathered to mourn the passing of our loved one and to share the finality of this, his life.

This is a tribute to a return soldier Phillip was HIV positive for 35 years. When he was diagnosed he was given months to live. He survived the war years when most of his friends died of horrific conditions and in many respects in appalling situations. Those were the days of discrimination, bigotry and the stark reality that life was and is very short.

As most of the people that know me can testify (only because its been the only topic of conversation for a couple of years) is that I wrote a book. I found it important and therapeutic to write down stories that have happened to me that I wanted to share with my nieces and nephews. Stories of food and people that have been important for me and my growth. Of course Phillip and Michael are in it.

I first met Phillip and Michael 16 years ago when I moved to South Australia. I met them at Cheltenham house a wonderful place (unfortunately recently closed) dedicated to working with HIV positive people who were either homeless, at risk of being or who were in need of respite.

Michael in those days was virtually non verbal one of the conditions he lived with was HIV dementia. The 2nd time I met them I'd mentioned that I lived in Northern rivers before coming here. That instantly got a reaction from Michael and we spoke at length about people we knew in common and were surprised we had never met each other. I looked at Philip and saw that he was very emotional

APPENDIX

tears streamed down his face. I asked him what the matter was? He said that I got to know more about Michael in the last 20 minutes than he had in the last 6 months.

I didn't realise it at the time but this was one of the only times I was ever going to see him cry. He had an exterior that was thicker than any wall Trump could build and he rarely shared emotions.

It was generally "Suck it up Princess"

I turned to him one time and said "I'm glad you acknowledge that I am royal"

Royal pain was his comment.

Watching changes over the years they were together I recall never seeing a more dedicated carer/partner relationship, that of Phillip's dedication to Michael. And in the chapter called "Don't Lie at Funerals" I have written about them. I had to write about this devoted loving relationship. Prior to meeting Michael, Phillip was not in a good place himself. So I believe for all that Phillip did for Michael, Michael gave in return by giving Phillip a reason to live.

Over the 8 years that they spent together, through all the tribulations, the absolute unchristian behaviour of some connections to Michael, we who were privileged to witness, saw a miracle. Michael became engaged and animated He had a joy of life that would not be there without Phillip. Michael would have died many years before without Phillip's intervention. Phillip gave Michael a quality of life that Michael's money or family did not give him. The irony is that "we" the unchristian were privy to the miracle and the Christian was oblivious to it. The Christian secured his stash of dollars and that is all.

APPENDIX

Phillip shared stories of Michael's life to me that will always haunt me. Stories that involve family decisions and "what was best" for Michael. The outcome of those decisions involved what we would classify today as torture but as a teenager he had electric shock treatments to cure the gay, and as an adult was committed to an institution where further violence and assault happened all under the banner of what was considered appropriate mental health processes.

Phillip saved the "family" millions of dollars with his 24 hour 7 days a week care and when Michael died more trauma was created by the christian where Phillip had to fight to get a roof over his head. Through all this Phillip kept his head high and didn't let the appalling behaviour get to him.

Phillip and Michael seemed to get sick at the same time as Mum and Dad which was incredibly challenging. Michael had a heart attack followed shortly by Dad having one. Then Mum was diagnosed with bowel cancer as was Phillip their operations were two days apart. I waited for him to recover and then jumped in the car to help mum after her operation. This happened on several occasions so towards the end I started telling him not to die on certain dates! Don't die on the same day as Aretha Franklin, don't die on my birthday, don't die at Christmas or New Year, don't die on Mum and dads 60th anniversary as it was he waited a day ! Their day was the 10th and it was the 11th he collapsed! I should have said don't die in the week of.........And as it was my birthday was two days ago He will continue to clash with other events and that's just the way he was!

APPENDIX

He thought he wouldn't make it to see the Alison Moyet concert or Grace Jones but he did! I'm glad he did!

Possibly the most emotional thing for me was that their relationship and the miracle that it was, will not be on the death certificate. Michael unfortunately died before defacto same sex relationships were recognised.

Phillip had secrets which were a pain in the arse for Betty and myself and I still have an issue or two with Phillip about that. This leads me onto Betty. Some people come into your life at the right time and place and none more finer to have by his side and my side is Betty Fawcett. 4 foot high but a tower of strength especially during the final few months and his hospitalisation.

He answered the door to Betty a few months ago. "Bugger Off you're not supposed to be here!"

Angela from RDNS was there I had made some "reason" to be there In reality we all were checking up on him. Betty he said, "I don't want you washing my jocks I want you to be there in the end." And that she was which included 2 x 24 hour shifts by his side during the week of his hospitalisation.

Unfortunately his care had some ups and downs at the RAH and that was particularly painful for us to watch. He'd handed over his life to us and said look after it. This included me doing my finest Joan Crawford impersonation to the nursing manager and doctors! I didn't shout I was cool, direct and blunt. I had Phillip as a mentor. We did look after him and I know I am proud of myself and of Betty that we were there to the end and more.

Meredith Brown always remember if its in your guts to

do something follow your stomach I can't thank you enough for your late night shift and having to deal with me snoring when I passed out.

Some may say Phillip had a sad life and in some respects it was but he was never found him sad. He could be angry, loud, judgemental, opinionated, verbally razor sharp and blunt.

He was a great friend and I loved him for that.

Au revior Phillip and thank you.

Betty our job is done xx

* * *

The War Years Interview, Radio Adelaide
Logan Bold interviewing Greg Kelly 2011

Can you explain what you call "The War Years"?

Almost from the time of coming out for me because I came out to Mum and Dad and that was very hard but beautiful because it ended up as Mum and Dad were wonderful human beings

A few months later Gay Plague was hitting the papers and that started some concern I had been going out to Gay pubs. Maybe within the next year or so Id been to a couple I started seeing men with gaunt looks maybe thinning hair, rashes on their faces, or hands flaky skin and you knew that it wasn't normal aging looks These people were sick

It didn't seem long before I went from observations in a pub to friends who needed lifts to the doctors getting sick to hospital and then people started to die.

APPENDIX

Very quickly we developed check lists that if someone was dying or had died suddenly we knew that we would have to go into the bedroom to remove movies toys make sure all the porn anything sexual was removed before you rang anyone so parents wouldn't discover the different collections. You had to make sure that it was done

It was a constant stream of cooking or getting food from the restaurants I was working at for friends who weren't or couldn't cook for themselves making sure everyone was fed.

It really surprised me one day I was about 19 or 20 and I came home to Mum and Dads and Mum said they had been watching this program on the impact of AIDS in Africa on kids and they wanted to help. Mum did some enquiries and found a house that was getting assistance from some nuns. It was set up by two guys John and Steve with the help of the nuns they set up St Francis House the first of its kind in the world for HIV positive people who had HIV drug and or alcohol related issues but then it got expanded to guys who were out of prison, transgender people anyone who was positive and had nowhere to go. One person was involved in a gender reassignment and was diagnosed and there fore the change just stopped half way through. In fact anybody who needed an operation didn't normally get it because the doctors wouldn't operate on positive people.

Mum and dad and I would go over to SFH we would help co-ordinate or just talk to people we would bring food and have a meal with the guys. There fore there was a base and a focus. Guys would live there they had a home, we would sometimes just talk, be a friend

We became friends. The 1st person who Mum Dad and I knew who died of AIDS was a gay man we didn't know for a long time yet he really affected us all he was the first of many to come

From that time I developed an extraordinary admiration for my parents and their capacity to give and we have till this day been close as ever.

The hardest thing I will ever have to do (after a connection to St Francis house of about three years) was to come out myself to Mum and dad as being positive it was the most painful thing I would ever have to do. The model of St Francis House was used as a guide by a Sister of the Mercy Order (Sister Margaret) and with the help of Centrecare the Dept of Health and the RDNS an Adelaide version was opened Cheltenham house. The day this was opened was the same day that Combination Therapy was introduced. The needs of positive people changed over night and the original plan for Cheltenham House had to adapt to those changing needs. Cheltenham House still is open to this day and survives as it has had to adapt but its focus is still on low level care for PLWHA's

In mid 1993 I had been given 6 months to live and I needed to tell Mum and Dad It was around the time that before combination therapy had come in I took a month or two to get my head around my diagnosis and then needed to tell them. They expected as did I that I was going to be buried in a short while but I wanted to make sure I lived longer than the 6 months I was given.

So the war years started dissipating about 96 or 97 that emergency stuff, blankets food things like that weren't as urgent. People were still dying sure but the needs of positive people started to change. The war years in particular were hands on, action was needed shoulders were needed; someone always needed some sort of attention, of some description making an appointment or organising a funeral.

APPENDIX

I always thought and believed that everyone was involved that everybody sort of was in their own way because what we were dealing with does, or will affect everybody but as I lived long enough what surprises me the most with the war years now, was that quite a few people I have met since still know nothing about this time. And here I was swamped in numbers of deaths; I attended over 80 funerals in a six or seven year period. It staggers me to think that we as a community have gone through an epidemic, a condition whatever you want to call it in numbers has surpassed the Spanish flu of the early 20th century more people have died to HIV/AIDS statistically (in gay world) than ww2 and yet we still have infections we still have ignorance and its almost passé to talk about being HIV positive It is staggering that I went through and many others went through the war years and now they seem to have been something we block out, block out of our minds and not really learn from How many have learnt from the war years?

I know I have learnt it's indelibly marked my consciousness and it will be part of me for the rest of my life. As to how may others I don't know and its affect on them seems minimal sometimes especially when you see bare backing promoted as some sort of romantic type of expression or even a right as opposed to a psycho Russian roulette game and that scares me because that we could go for a second war.

Do I miss the galvanized community?

There was a certain camaraderie that developed to the people that were involved an extraordinary capacity to love care and give. And through the war years I saw the greatest that humanity has to offer. People came out of the wood work to assist. What can I do? What can I get? And those who would give time and time again these were the best people I have ever met.

I know they are out there.

Those years are linked intrinsically to the so called gay agenda of today

Those years were a catalyst for things like GMH women's health HIV research and other virus research for so many things that have benefited society broadly. Viruses were a theory before HIV they had never been photographed or studied at all. In certain ways I might say that I do miss it I don't miss the suffering but the absolute respect that I have for many people that are nameless souls in our world who assisted in the crisis.

I think today in many respects there is ambivalence about those years

Nothing irritates me more than gay white males in comfortable jobs who are HIV negative who say I'm so over HIV. I know the beauty pageants the Mr leathers and others where contestants are told not to mention HIV.

Would you say to a Vietnam vet I'm so over talking about Agent Orange side effects?

Would you say to a survivor of a concentration camp I'm over war talk?

Would you say it to anyone who had seen armed conflict to shut up?

I would think that it would be a stupid insensitive person that would say that to a person who has been raped, run over or traumatized in some horrific way to silence their own grief.

I find it amazing that we as a community have the capacity would turn on our heroes virtually someone who

APPENDIX

has been pos for 15, 20 30 years is a hero to me for surviving.

As far as I'm concerned you might as well urinate on the shrine of remembrance when

That's how I feel when I hear that appalling disdain like "I'm over AIDS!"

I was reading a famous gay HIV historian Larry Kramer who has written a really bad article with many "they's" they aren't looking after us etc. Far too many generalizations to have much meaning but just as nasty as the so called born again Christians

And I have to say that "They" can be the gay negative men who say I'm so over it

Or the men who don't know they are positive and are too gutless to get tested and have unsafe sex and then there is the extended friends and families of these people who cant or wont approach the subject with these sexually active people. They are all included in the "they's" and these men are as bad as the screwed up Christians.

We can be our own worst enemies as a community today

Getting diagnosed was the greatest cosmic kick in the arse that I will ever have. It was the defining moment in my life.

I was starting to look at my spirituality during this time and was reading Louise Hay and Marianne Williamson and others. I recall going "oh yeh sexual guilt" being a bit cynical and went onto doing some pretty hard soul searching and I believe that it would be a very hard task to find a gay man who has been through a religious upbringing or has religion in their background who doesn't have some guilt associated with their desires stemming from a religious experience. It can be a really good cultural Petri dish for self loathing.

It made me stop and look at my life and see where my life was heading.

What are the things that I want to make sure I want to tick off the bucket list if I do die in 6 months?

I saw films that I wanted to see

I read books I wanted to read

Things I wanted to do

Disney cartoons I never saw as a kid

And I think I have been living life like that ever since.

I challenged the guilt in my head, the shame and whatever negative aspect associated with my sexuality

It was the catalyst for me to change

Who knows with hindsight had I not been diagnosed what or who I might be? I think I'd be a stressed out heavy drinking chef that burnt out by 40

I'm glad I'm not that person I love the person I am today

I wouldn't be that person I am today without those three little letters

It's where you put it in your head that matters

It doesn't rule my life

Life rules my life

*　*　*

Candlelight Vigil – November 30th 2011

On the 28th Of November I celebrated entering my 20th year of being HIV positive. I celebrate because I was told I had 6 months to live and the one thing I wanted to do when I was told that news was to prove that doctor wrong!!

So many of my friends for whatever reason did not

make it when that bone was pointed at them and they were told they were going to die. They did.

During this time a lot suffered intolerably and I call these years from the late 80's till mid 90's the war years. I lived through some things that were just enough for one lifetime.

I don't know why I was one of the ones left standing that in itself has been an issue with me what is clinically referred to as survivor guilt.

HIV showed me extremes of humanity.

I believe I really started my life journey I was awoken to life with HIV and the deaths of so many and also the amazing way in how so many people responded to the crisis. I witnessed a father who spat on his son's grave because of what he died from and what he was.

I was honoured to have my parents who in the late 1980's, started to do volunteer work with positive and drug and alcohol affected mainly men. In a house in Melbourne that was a fore runner to Adelaide's Cheltenham place. And on a note of history those of you that have been in the fight for such a long time I urge you now to write down your history. As PLC's become PLSA'S and other institutions fade and become something else it is imperative to get as accurate an account of this time as possible by as many of you that are still here because someone else will get the opportunity to write it and they will be writing from their perspective.

HIV was the greatest cosmic kick in the behind I will ever have and the greatest tool I will ever be given. I never thought about my mortality or even what sort of impression I was leaving on this planet. Which is a pity in itself (but also a golden opportunity) that it does take a death sentence for one to really get real about one's life

Some of the questions I asked myself after diagnosis were

If I did die what are the things that I would have regrets about??

Are there people that I am withholding apologies or niceties from? Are there people I haven't told I love them?

Are there books movies or places that I want to see?

Are there things that need doing?

What sort of impact have I actually made on this planet and to the people around me?

These questions were my starting blocks for I believe the strong foundation I have built with the help of so many people both on this side of the mortal coil as well as the other side they all have guided me for the last twenty years.

I recently finished two diplomas in community welfare and one of the things that was incredibly confronting for me but very powerful was a lecturer who hooked her leg in a chair and dragged the chair across the floor saying see that chair that's all your dead friends. How do you think they would feel if they were being dragged around like this??

It took a while but I do believe I have been able to let the pain and suffering go as I do know that I will always remember the most amazing times the most amazing laughter from all my dead friends. They like my parents came into my life and honoured me with their presence they set the example.

I can't dwell on how my friends died because I would end up in a dark place I have to accept what happened and learn from that.

And what are the things I have learnt?

Every single day is precious

Every word I say and action I act has power

Life is far too short to waste but if you do waste time

make sure its on a fabulous comfy couch with some fantastic chocolate and tell yourself that time out is just as important as time hooked into the system.

I believe I am responsible for everything I do in this life and everything that happens to me.

I was privileged to be in this fight and now I can see the impact it has had on the younger generation

I have been a carer and have been cared for

I have been a guinea pig and I have benefited from my brothers and sisters who took horrible doses of medication so science could learn and I could live.

HIV is not all my life but it is an integral part.

If ever history decides to forget this lesson I feel that we would be doomed to repeat the terror.

I continue to be inspired with life and at the back of my mind on days when I'm despondent or at times like this where emotion is raw I use the RSL's motto in honour and praise to all that have helped me be here today

From my doctors and medical staff, parents, family and friends and those that put a smile on my face for a brief minute or two

LEST WE FORGET

* * *

Premiere of Why Wouldn't You? Mercury Cinema 2013
My film acting debut

G'day my name is Greg Kelly and I was diagnosed as HIV positive over twenty years ago. In those days I was given a life expectancy of 6 months. When that happened I was determined to prove the doctor wrong and here I am 20 years later. Needless to say mine has not been an isolated journey. I have always had the love and support of my parents, extended family and friends. Something that is still quite a rarity in modern Australia.

In 1986 and for about 5 years after my parents and I did volunteer work at a half way house for men who had major drug and alcohol issues and who were dying rather horrible deaths. My parents became surrogate parents to many men that had been rejected by their own families. They were scared lonely souls that had been ostracised by not only their families and friends but in many circumstances the government institutions and the law, religion police NGO social services like the Salvos and even by some members of the gay community. It was for me a war in those days. I stopped counting after 80 funerals.

I have often volunteered for things since those days and as the issues around HIV/AIDS have changed for services and individuals so have the jobs that have been needed to be done. Being involved in this project and another previous project with ACSA and gay men's health promotional issues is my way of continuing doing something for the community. And at the same time I am learning new skills from computers, to writing and script development.

After all this time I believe I have a voice and have lived experience that I can bring to the table. The issues around young men not getting tested are complex but in many cases have more to do with stigma and fear than any other explanation. Not that I'm saying fear isn't real, but one would have thought after nearly 30 years of knowing about HIV that stigma around sexual expression would have dissipated. Unfortunately statistics don't support this assumption of mine.

APPENDIX

Statistics need to be blended with the human element when doing a project like this. As the virus and issues around it have changed so have the messages that need to be delivered to target groups. Sero discordant relationships, CALD issues, other cultural or religious issues or negotiating sexual situations for those that don't identify are but a few of the more contemporary topics that face workers.

Without community involvement in campaigns like this one the end result can miss the target altogether. We as a society have some real presenting issues that will and do affect our young people. It's a tragedy that we have come so far that there are pills that can keep the virus at bay but many of our young people have not benefited from the advancement in empowered life knowledge.

Whatever the reasons for this I feel it part of my social duty to keep beating the drum.

I do hope you enjoy our effort and more importantly be able to use this resource and consider it of value to target groups x Thank You

* * *

Presentation to HHPP, World AIDS day 2011

(HIV and Hep C Programs and Policies section of Department of Health the most ignorant of people sometimes)

Hi I'm here to talk about my involvement with this project.

I have to preface my few minutes with some facts On Nov 28th I celebrated entering my 20th year of being told I had six months to live

As I state in the film the period of the late 80's to early 90's I refer to as The War Years. They were for me a very much hands on, get involved time capsule. There were meals to be made people to be taken to appointments and of course the organising and or attending funerals. Many of those that had passed died in extreme health circumstances as well as extreme family situations. So many farewells for a lot of men the only family they had were a few friends and maybe some workers. In some circumstances when families were involved if they weren't angry at there son they were contesting wills and winning, forcing partners to sell homes and possessions seemingly seconds after their sons had died. That was the level of involvement a lot of families had.

I recently finished two diplomas in community welfare one in counselling and the other in mental health. I have done some projects on the organisations you fund, how funding applications come in and how things happen. So believe me the honour to speak in front of you all is not lost on me.

As the times have changed and the needs of PLWHA's have changed it must be difficult to keep relevant when needs change dramatically. Case in point the day Cheltenham Place opened was the same day combination therapy was released. We all know the dramatic impact that had on peoples lives so an establishment that opened with the idea of really caring for people in their last days of dying almost over night has to change its focus.

I mention this because in many respects this funding model seems to work but with a condition like HIV that has changed dramatically over the last 30 years sometimes doesn't catch up. Or was relevant 6 months a year ago but has changed and might miss the point when funding process plays out.

As a positive person when you are poor and in bad health and life is difficult it's fantastic to be able to count on

APPENDIX

a service like the HIVE at the PLC or when available, to have some financial assistance through the BGF/Red Ribbon Fund for your medication. When the blessing of good health arises it is hard to not see the handouts as just that and maybe it would be great to have something that will give me some skills or maybe deal with underlying issues that are keeping me poor.

This project has been incredibly empowering It has been a multi levelled skill development workshop that I believe could be taken to any community setting from Indigenous to newly arrived people from the aged to the healthy.

Personally I have done many projects at VAC, ACON Nthn. Rivers, QUAC, and ACSA. It has been hard to walk away after finishing some projects without feeling like a powerless victim. It does appear that as a client if I behave the worst I will get the loudest response.

I have had two employment periods at ACSA of which I had some extremely challenging positive clients. I've met and seen some people with really challenging behaviour in my normal life. I think I've had a decent look a lot of the issues facing positive people.

What this project has allowed for me; and I believe and its what I have in common with all the groups I've mentioned, is the importance of telling our story. The ability to have a record of what has been significant in our lives, that is in our voices, from our thoughts and pens, it's extremely alluring.

When the project was first mentioned to me I relished the opportunity to tell "My Story".

What developed was I had more than one story to tell. So the offer was given to do two which was great. And of course I could go 3 4 5 etc. But I digress.

APPENDIX

Firstly there was writing the story then fine tuning the story and being aware that it needed to be said in a few minutes.

The collection of images either still or moving to match dialogue was another powerful tool as well as images that said something without dialogue

Then the computer skills involved in getting that process organised.

Putting finished projects onto discs etc or even just the transfer of files from one position on the computer to another was fantastic.

These have all been skills that I have been able to develop through this project.

I have also been given the opportunity to have as much or as little input as desired. We were given the option to not put our faces on or even do our voices which was really a liberating thing.

Greg's Sermon

Is something that I am really proud of, never had any training in any of these mediums. The message that I want to portray is, guilt and shame can make you do and can be the reason you allow other people to do things to you, things you may not want to happen.

No matter what anyone says to you when the person you are going to have an intimate connection with doesn't want to protect you and them REMEMBER ONE THING- do you want to be undeniably connected to a drug company for the rest of your life? Long term multiple medication use has major effects on the quality of your life. Some deal with it better than others but do you really need to deal with it?

APPENDIX

I showed a non finished version on a retreat I volunteered to cater at in Northern Rivers to about 40 positive men of diverse age and cultures and got enormous positive response from them. A few of the young men in their twenties told me that if they had seen this message ten years ago this would have changed their lives. Due to the fact there were people from Sydney and country NSW as well as Queensland at the retreat clients have been asking ACON and positive groups in Queensland for a similar project for them.

I was asked by an older man who helps run the QLD GLBTIQ archives held at the State library in Brisbane for in particular "Greg's Sermon" because of its relevance and directness.

At the launch at Feast of positive stories I was overwhelmed with the response from everyone so were Mum and Dad who came over for the event. I entered this into the Bear Film festival and received high praise. I'm intending on entering any film festival I can find.

I was asked and did write an article for Talkabout about the process which is the NSW HIV magazine and in which of course I put the links on. If you look on line it should be available today.

I have put it on two different Private Facebook HIV positive groups to high praise. I'm very aware that I have a strong message that is really powerful

Another amazing quality about this project is finding my voice.

At the launch at Feast there was conversation with Feast people, several international performers and workers like Rob from SHINE and Logan from the AIDS Council and Suzi at PLSA about where to from here?

Television has been mentioned in particular late night

APPENDIX

RAGE or Andrew Dentons television shows The Gruen Transfer, Hungry Beast.

At the end of the launch the audience was asked how can they help get this message out.

I now ask you.

In these days of social media Safe Sex messages don't seem to be apparent or seen. Let's face it who looks at posters anymore?

This is a safe sex message from a community member I can say things that the bodies you fund can't or get stopped from saying. I own this message.

I believe my message has already started to impact and I believe you can help me impact more lives.

There has not been a national campaign since the days of the Grim reaper.

Because the media was confined to television, newspapers and radio No message could have the same impact that the Grim reaper had then, today because of social media, internet and the like. Today the objective is to get tweeted about or get on you tube.

I'm prepared to put my face out there to assist in safety messages in any way I can and to do it as best as I can I need you to help.

You are a state body that must have connections to federal bodies and organisations. I urge you to assist in any way you can. The organisations you fund who are working on the coal face know there is power in being blunt and direct to the youth target group. And it must be directed to the social media phenomenon here is an opportunity for a project stemming from SA that potentially can go global.

And the exquisite beauty of this Positive stories project for me is that there can be messages made cheaply having

APPENDIX

maximum impact directed at community members made by community members.

*　*　*

Speech for Positive Stories, 2011

Getting involved in a workshop was fantastic

The skills or lack of was not an issue in the process which I really enjoyed.

Everyone came with different ideas and different levels of skill. To be given a chance to learn new skills was there and the capacity to take hold of the reigns as well as standing back and maybe just doing a bit of directing here and there.

The priority was to tell our story and to get it onto a format.

I am still recovering from "Holding the Man" a play that brought back a flood of memories. There are coincidences in that book with Mum dad and my lives. The priest that buried John was sitting at the table when I told mum and Dad we knew many people referenced in the book

And seeing the play reminded me again of how extraordinary my parents actually are. Mum and Dad made friends and were carers for, men from all sorts of gay lifestyles including those with drug habits or who had been in prison or who were dancers from the Australian Ballet but men that were dying of some terrible conditions. I felt a compulsion to share my parents with you all because I am extremely proud of Margaret and Vin. I recently finished two diplomas in community welfare and was exposed to an enormous amount of issues in our world. I'm not saying that bad stuff doesn't happen to good people (and I ain't saying I haven't been a little evil in my time!) but when challenges have arisen in my life its been vital to know that I have a steady and loving relationship with family which can and does get me through to where I need to be.

I know that I as a gay man am some what of a rarity too many men I have known have suffered intolerably at the hands of family.

I have thoroughly enjoyed this process and I can suggest it as a therapeutic tool for any workers out there who deal in community issues. Everyone has a voice and everyone has a story to tell. And everyone's story is important including mine

* * *

Stigma and Discrimination: A Personal Story, 2012

Since Logan asked me to do this I have pondered on the topic and the closer I have come tonight memories of things that have happened to me have popped in to say hello.

This hasn't been particularly easy bringing up the past.

Growing up in the Catholic school system and being I'll admit a Nancy boy I learnt first hand about discrimination. From primary and secondary the trip in the playground was backed by Jesus because Jesus didn't allow or like poofters either.

I was diagnosed nearly twenty years ago.

I with my parents had done volunteer work before that, with positive people in the mid to late 80's and early 90's we got a first hand lesson in societal discrimination My

APPENDIX

mother had invited five positive men to her fiftieth, one particularly unwell man in a wheelchair. Some guests were lets say confronted. In those days doctors refused to operate on positive people priests refused to bury, even the Salvos weren't hospitable we saw this.

I tried to get insurance when I had a restaurant and had responded to one of the questions about so called high risk behaviour that yes I was a man who had sex with men. The second questionnaire that came back included questions of the type of what sexual behaviour I participated in how many and all manner of other questions. I wouldn't get covered if I didn't respond to the questions. Needless to say I didn't get covered.

Another company Alliance (who insured the third Reich) refused to give me comprehensive car insurance because I was on a pension. I wouldn't be on the pension without HIV.

This sort of institutionalised discrimination reminds me as well of being in a suburban hospital in pain I cannot describe for five days I had been on morphine and six doctors and specialists were coming in and telling me something different about removing spleens and kidneys and other body parts. I screamed at the head nurse I wouldn't speak to another doctor until they all came at once. They finally did this and asked all of them for the 100th time had they all checked the medication side effects looking them in the eye they all looked at the "lackey" doctor who ran out got out his MiMMs and came back with Indinivir side effects. They all knew better than me or so they thought!

I believe that in many ways all health bodies or institutions are failing to reach out to educate other community sectors as well as the general public. Educational specific sexual content information is so limited if targeted campaigns fail to appear because someone in the health department doesn't like what they see. This creates ignorance.

The main sort of discrimination that has hurt though is the inter personal discrimination from gay men. Briefly I have been spat at assaulted verbally and physically I have had to walk into a packed gay bar naked because I had ventured upstairs with a gent who asked me up for the night. I disclosed way before going upstairs I was positive, when it got down to the deed I grabbed condoms and that's when I was thrown out naked.

I have been in a room of gay men when there was a few dollars being spoken about what to do with it I said we are meeting at the AIDS council why don't we donate it to the wellness fund. The response came back You AIDS people are all the same always asking for money.

It seems in gay world to talk about being positive or issues relating is passé.

What really can upset me today is terminology in gay world where words like clean has crept into the internet cruise sites and local vernacular in particular websites like bbrt where unsafe sexual practices are promoted. I don't know as a positive man who has always been told unsafe sex is illegal immoral etc just how to deal with bbrt? Gents on these sites seem to believe that calling themselves undetectable will make sure they don't get or give any disease? There appears to be no moral or legal issues with giving and getting potential diseases of all types. Medicine started the use of this word and possibly now to its detriment. There are also men saying they are negative but having received on numerous occasions don't care what status they are. Why does it seem, to get HIV and if you want to live, take meds for the rest of your life, not so bad? Being totally connected to a drug company for ever? Why is that not bad? These are not random profiles there is a considerable number. Where does the dilemma moral or ethical end and finish? The idea of the bug chaser where's the personal responsibility where's the institutional responsibility start and end? Are the institutions making themselves present on these websites? Is it up to the institutions or is it personal freedom? If so to me I can be charged and put in jail (as in the most vocal of the Sth Australian transmission cases) for these things and maybe others wont for the same thing.

This whole area I feel is a mine field of so called moral and freedom issues to me one of the only campaigns that has come out of that invoked some sort of personal responsibility was the Grim Reaper and that is just sad.

The use of AIDS the word today is an anathema to me because AIDS council and bodies through out the country don't see what they saw 10 or 15 years ago. They are doing very different jobs possibly not connected to AIDS I believe its continuing use creates stereotyping and even mottos "A future free of HIV" is technically at this present stage a future by implication without me!

I wouldn't be who I am without the life I have lived I am troubled by this new world and feel that having gone through one war I appear to be looking at another in the future. If being positive isn't a big thing, how has this message got out? Funny nothing's a big deal ....until diagnoses.

* * *

Digital Story Telling Project
Article printed in Talkabout, a HIV Magazine, 2011

APPENDIX

G'day my name is Greg Kelly and I have lived with HIV for (oh shit soon to be 20 years!) I've lived in four states now and I feel I have seen the "HIV" industry change and adapt as the needs of positive people have changed. Some good changes some not so.

I have been asked to share my thoughts about the process of making a digital story. The end result- a three minute video clip, a type of experience, sharing a story that is relevant to me. In other words, me talking about me, what's not to like about that?? (he he)

The project was funded by a program with the AIDS Council of SA and Feast (SA's Queer Festival). I got involved from the start as it seemed that I would get a few new skills. This is possibly one of the few projects that I have been involved with, put on by an AIDS council, where I have finished the project feeling empowered as opposed to sad or sort of feeling like a victim.

The empowerment is similar to the feeling when leaving one of those fabulous Northern Rivers retreats! It's like a sense of having gone on a wonderful journey. I have a tangible thing that I can do something with. I have actually learnt something that I can apply in other parts of my life!

I've had an interesting "walk" around some things that even my old computer can do and learnt about what some other programs not on my computer can do.

I also really enjoyed having a space to tell my story. I appreciate the acknowledgment from governing bodies (in the shape of funding) that I actually have a story to tell.

The process of formulating a story and being able to write it, refine it, get images that go with the text and then to tell it, record it and have music put to my voice which I have to admit makes me feel a little bit of a "star" in my own

APPENDIX

lunch box that is! Essentially it has made me laugh and I hope others will too.

The importance of telling my story I believe is that I appear to have lived through an experience that for one moment in time was one of the key topics of the news, was happening everywhere (or so it seemed) and I was a soldier in the what I call the "Love Army". The people that came from "nowhere" that were mothers, fathers, nuns (defying Melbourne's bishop), some priests, they were brothers, sisters, aunts and uncles friends they were gay lesbian bi sexual tri anything people, or were just people who saw that there was suffering and they offered a hand.

At the same time as this an HIV positive 5 year old girl was deported out of Australia and forced to live in New Zealand (could such a thing happen today?). The days where the blood bank didn't want to test all the blood they were given because of cost –(discrimination still exists against gay men), Salvos weren't so friendly and they had issues accommodating or offering proper services to PLWHA as we became known as. In those days of course we were known as "AIDS victims" and we were to be feared, pitied and in many cases judged as filth by the mainstream of society "who were worse than lower forms of life because they either did unspeakable acts with each other or stuck needles in their arms -They deserve it - God's wrath!".

On the opposite side became a fire in the belly of men and women that became ACT-UP and similar organisations where an almost revolutionary politics swept into gay world. In my perception it took HIV/AIDS to be the impetus which triggered a lot of reforms on equality and same sex relationship status that are demanded today.

Some images of the war will be with me always those of my dear friends with horrific conditions and yet at the same time I witnessed the best that humanity has to offer these people raged against this crushing virus that took so many from us. These caring people assisted those in need, in so many ways and in many cases took the place of family during the last months or years up until and at the time and place of death.

HIV certainly doesn't define me but I have to admit like a returned serviceman it takes up a part of and always will be a part of my story.

And so now in 2011 heading to 2012 HIV/AIDS related issues not making headlines or not being in the public eye as it was (way back then).

Who is to blame for increases in infections? Who is at fault? Is there anyone or anything to blame? Where is the system failing? Is there any part of bureaucracy that has failed? Could it be the religious right high jacking the argument by not permitting proper health education to happen in many religious based and government schools? Where is the line in the sand on personal responsibility and negligence by others?

I am responsible for every single thing that I do AND if I want to get a bit Louise Hay on you I am responsible for everything that happens to me as well. Random acts can be just that, but it is how I react to the act, that is the most important thing. Life truly has sucked in many ways for me if it hadn't of sucked I probably wouldn't know or be able to appreciate the fabulous people and things that also have come my way during my life. I hasten to add I am saying this at the old man age of 46 and with a bit of hind sight.

I have a quote by someone called Epictetus on my front door. I see it every time I enter and leave as does everyone who comes into my front door.

APPENDIX

"People are disturbed not by things, but by the views they take of them".

Me Mum and Dad
Is a testimony to my parents who had their number four child come out to them as a seventeen year old and a month or two later "Gay Plague hits Melbourne" were the headlines of the Sun newspaper. Margaret and Vincent got involved in volunteer work with HIV positive people at a place called St Francis House, the first of its kind in Australia. It accommodated HIV positive people mainly with drug and alcohol issues. Mum and Dad mixed with effeminate gay men, masculine gay men, Trans genders, people just out of prison and people who used intravenously, all colours.

Mum starred in a Channel 7 documentary the opening scene showing a man injecting heroin. The first time this had ever been shown on television possibly in the world.

She was interviewed on commercial radio several times and has authored articles published in Australian Catholic newspapers telling of hers and Dad's experiences with HIV positive people.

Mum and Dad keep telling me they are just normal people (whatever that is) I know from my experiences of friends and the wider GLBTIQQ communities they are far from normal and this is the least I can do to pay homage to them for their courage, support and strength.

Please check out Rainbow family tree website set up by Sonja Vivenne and if you have a story or want to tell a story in this format then I urge you to try you'll be surprised who just really is interested in something you have to say. The site can show you how to do the process or hassle your local AIDS council to set up what we have done here in South

Australia. I believe that it is a really therapeutic thing to do, to tell your story. You've got nothing to lose. Take a few moments to check out our stories we all have something to say.

The videos are available at: Vimeo.com/gregkelly

* * *

The Winsome Hotel, 2012
(Piece added to a collation of recollections of The Winsome Hotel being collated by University students at Southern Cross Uni)

It was through a mutual friend that Peter and I met. He had been in Lismore and thought he had walked into the other pub down the road looking for a cheap meal. He was told by the barman that if he wanted something to eat "The kitchens out the back and could he cook something for him to?"

It became pretty obvious the pub was having a lull in popularity. Peter spoke to John and John introduced me to Peter. Within a fortnight we seemed to have taken over the running of a pub kitchen. My aim was to just have a space to organise a party or two to help fundraise for the local HIV community. Being a member of that community and having received benefits, I wanted to do my bit to give back.

Within days it appeared we had a business, we then decided to have an opening party. I wanted to make sure we had a few weeks before this party to "run in" this new thing we were doing. During this time we CLEANED! We also opened the restaurant and started serving meals.

The kitchen was filthy as was so many of the rooms

upstairs! Dining room was full of cobwebs and dust. Crappy curtains were dust ridden and some just crumbled at touch heavy with years of nicotine in the air. Such discoveries though! I found little corners and nooks in stair wells that were full of crockery and all sorts of kitchen stuff that seemed to have been put away a century ago (or at least 10 years!)

I did the invites and called the party "Stick me to your fridge!" The cover of the invite was of me, naked except for my chef's hat and a strategically placed fry pan and I think a sprig of rosemary in my mouth! It was my 34th birthday party a fund raiser for the HIV wellness fund and the opening of "Two Bridges restaurant".

There are moments in my life when I look back and just am always humbled as to the out pouring of generosity. This was one of those times. We had a jazz band up stairs in the dining room, late afternoon opening out on the balcony where amazing fabrics were draped from to the ground. When welcomes and band were done upstairs, we descended to ground level to enter the party that had already begun. So about 200 people hit another 200 and the party took off.

There were eight DJs who donated their time to the event. The sound system was provided by a friend we had male, female, Trans artists of the burlesque variety. The lighting was donated by some wonderful men. The building had those big movie lights that flood lit the building. We had all the "stars" of the community! They know who they are, as many costumes were made for that night as a Troppo Fruits dance!

We had fireworks! At 1 am we had organised a glitter bomb to go off. The music stopped I ran out into the middle of the back verandah (no longer there) which was a dance floor I ripped open my shirt as the lights flashed and the explosion happened covering me in silver glitter. Unfortunately I had my mouth open as well, thus getting a mouth full! It went through the boards onto the dance floor downstairs that was set up as a more techno space with fluoro stuff everywhere and where it rained glitter for hours.

My father arrived as a surprise from Melbourne with my sisters and their families from the coast. Dad read a speech that Mum had written that was spoken about for years. There wasn't a dry eye in the house. Dad said incredulously "Do you know all these people?" My reply was well yes most! I was running all night offering food playing host and just loving every moment of this extraordinary event. We had just over 600 people. I had 5 birthday cakes one which included a paper replica hand made of the Hotel. I had that for years but it finally died in a flood!

What was the restaurant downstairs became a chill out area where some of the older people relaxed away from the loud music. We raided everyone's gardens before the event to get some lavish floral displays that were quite incredible. The community of GLBTIQ's creative inspiration team came to town and did the Hotel a makeover!! We organised local artists to hang work throughout the hotel. There were installations of amazing things I have little recollection of particular things though I just knew that it was fabulous and it all just seemed to happen!

The front bar had a cocktail bar as well as the main bar and that was always full and that had another sound system set up. We even organised a pokie machine that had a drag queen and you had to get gold stilettos in a row.

The stables out the back had a good clean out of all the rats and other creatures that hadn't been bothered in years. Again lighting and hay bales were added to give it a chill

APPENDIX

feel and was quite popular with the boys that night. The police arrived with some noise complaints so eventually at about 2 o'clock we took the party mainly in doors and the last left at about 6 am.

My dear friend Alan made me very proud a day or two before the opening of the party he climbed the hotel up to the flag pole which had a very raggedy Australian flag. It was no more than a bit of cloth he replaced this with the rainbow flag that flew for the first time over Lismore from such a height!

I still say today 14 years later that I have had the best birthday party I will ever have it truly was a magnificent event and it is still talked about today. I'm very proud of my connection to this place, in a way I helped create something amazing and to this day I and the Hotel and a few other people have gone down in the mythology of the Northern Rivers!

There was a makeover at the Winsome Hotel that shook Lismore into the night and the next morning - all for my birthday!! And we raised nearly $1500 on the night for the HIV wellness fund.

ACKNOWLEDGMENTS

I would like to thank everyone mentioned in this book and also a lot of people who aren't. Good, bad and indifferent if I have encountered you in my life, you have been part of the experience that has culminated in who I am today. That is alive and grateful for that!

To Merri Brown for such dedication, at correcting all my spelling and grammar, for the amazing task of proof reading nine drafts and for believing in this project from your first read which has been an integral part of its completion; my undying thanks.

To Grant Burford for "Greg's Eye's", and "Mum and Dad". Shane Duniam for the "Sea Scapes" all of your art pieces inspire and delight. Thank you

To Raymond Zada your skill in the design of the cover. And Liza Reynolds for styling me! Thank you

To Mum, Dad, my brothers and sisters and to my nieces and nephews this is for you.

Margaret, Vincent, Libby, Dave, Bernard, Jenny, Paul, Leanne, Majella, Daryl, Matthew, Trudi, Benjamin, Aaron,

Joshua, Samuel, Lucas, Damian, Jordan, Gemma, Aidan, Finn, Tara and Jayden - shine bright xx

Love your Son, Brother and Uncle - Greg

RECIPES

CHAPTER ONE

- Nana Young's Quince Jam and Paste - pg. 2
- Shane's Hainan Chicken - pg. 14
- Preparing a Bird for Cooking - pg. 40
- Clement's Hainan Method - pg. 40
- Beef Stock and Game Stocks - pg. 41
- Fish Stock - pg. 42
- Vegetable Stock - pg. 43
- Miso Soup - pg. 44
- My Asian-Inspired Broth - pg. 45
- Prawn or Shellfish Stock - pg. 46

CHAPTER TWO

- Method for Herb Butter - pg. 51
- Base Recipe Sable Biscuits - pg. 52

RECIPES

- Almond Bread - pg. 54
- Meringues - pg. 55
- Anzacs Biscuits - pg. 56
- Biscotti - pg. 57
- Brandy Snaps - pg. 58
- Brandy Snap Baskets - pg. 58
- Cornets - pg. 60
- Crostolli - pg. 61
- Marcella Hazan – Chiacchiere Della Nonna – Sweet Pastry Fritters - pg. 62
- Dutch Biscuits - pg. 63
- Gingerbread - pg. 64
- Royal Icing - pg. 65
- Haakons - pg. 66
- Melting Moments - pg. 66
- Lemon Filling - pg. 67
- Yo-Yos - pg. 68
- Shortbread - pg. 68
- Orange Biscuits - pg. 68
- Chocolate Fudge Cookies - pg. 69
- Ciambella - pg. 70
- Almond Numbers pg. 71
- Almond Number 2 (no-bake) - pg. 72
- Gluten Free Peanut Numbers - pg. 73
- Susie's Vegan Numbers - pg. 73

CHAPTER THREE

- Ivana's Bread - pg. 80
- Muffins - pg. 82
- Soda Bread - pg. 83
- Hot Onion Bread - pg. 84

RECIPES

- Belle's Damper - pg. 85
- Banana Bread - pg. 87
- Brioche - pg. 95
- Crayfish Mousseline - pg. 95
- Bisque Sauce - pg. 96
- Plain Batter - pg. 97
- Choux Pastry - pg. 98
- Tempura Batter - pg. 98
- Flourless Chocolate Cake - pg. 100
- Similar (but with a touch of flour) Chocolate Cake - pg. 101
- Roast Beef - pg. 113
- Gravy Jus - pg. 115

CHAPTER FOUR

- Passionfruit Sorbet (Machine Version) - pg. 130
- Sorbet (By Hand or Mix-Master) - pg. 131
- Ivana's Pasta - pg. 142
- Ivana's Cannelloni Filling - pg. 144
- Spinach and Fetta Filling - pg. 145
- Polenta and Vegetable Soufflé - pg. 146
- Thai-Inspired Red Curry Sauce - pg. 149
- Annesley's Chicken Korma - pg. 152
- Annesley's Burryiani - pg. 153
- Pickled Sprouts - pg. 154
- Cous-Cous - pg. 156
- Rissoles – Chicken, Beef, Lamb, Kangaroo - pg. 156

RECIPES

CHAPTER FIVE

- Rehydration Fluid - pg. 163
- Vinaigrette - pg. 167
- Ginger and Sesame Dressing - pg. 168
- A Bit of a Tartare Dressing - pg. 169
- Asian-Inspired Dressing - pg. 170
- Mango Sauce - pg. 171
- Great Marinade for Red Meat - pg. 171
- Beurre Blanc for Two - pg. 172
- Oysters San Francisco - pg. 173
- A Vague Curry Sauce - pg. 174
- Thai Beef Salad Dressing - pg. 175
- Herb Paste - pg. 176
- Crème Anglaise - pg. 176
- Crème Patisserie - pg. 177

CHAPTER SIX

- Best Chocolate Fudge - pg. 190
- Lemon Cordial - pg. 191
- Marshmallows - pg. 192
- Pear Honey or Sauce - pg. 193
- Date Chutney - pg. 193
- Mango Chutney - pg. 194
- Mum's Chocolate Crunch - pg. 195
- Mum's Raspberry Shortcake - pg. 196
- Mum's Apple Batter Cake - pg. 196
- Engadine - pg. 197
- Strawberry Flummery pg. 198

RECIPES

CHAPTER SEVEN

- Chocolate Whiskey Raisin Cake - pg. 207
- Joanne's Apricot Sherbet - pg. 214
- Muesli - pg. 214
- My Chocolate Pudding - pg. 216
- Mum's Boiled Chocolate Cake - pg. 217
- Shane's Beetroot and Chocolate Cake - pg. 218
- Fudge Chocolate Brownies - pg. 219
- Dining Room Chocolate Cake - pg. 219
- Chocolate Marquis - pg. 220
- Chocolate and Macadamia Torte - pg. 221
- Mississippi Mud Cake - pg. 223
- Chicken and Vegetable Soup - pg. 226
- Risotto - pg. 228
- Orange and Cardamom Jelly - pg. 229

CHAPTER EIGHT

- Mum's Cheesecake - pg. 239
- Baked Cheesecake - pg. 239
- Auntie Bess's Sponge - pg. 240
- Auntie Shelia's Plain Cake - pg. 241
- Bread and Butter Pudding - pg. 242
- Citrus Tart - pg. 243
- Lemon Butter - pg. 243
- Lemon Delicious - pg. 244
- Mum's Nut Loaf - pg. 245
- Mum's Pavlova - pg. 246
- Nana Young's Fruit Cake - pg. 246
- Fruit Mince - pg. 248

RECIPES

- Panforte - pg. 249
- Middle Eastern Orange Cake pg. 250
- Fig and Pecan Pie - pg. 251
- Apricot Tofu Cake - pg. 251
- Sticky Date Pudding - pg. 252
- Summer Pudding - pg. 253

CHAPTER NINE

- Tapenade - pg. 264
- Hommos - pg. 265
- My Babaganoush - pg. 265
- Salmon Rillettes - pg. 266
- Samosa Filling - pg. 267
- Samosa Pastry - pg. 267
- Mussels - pg. 268
- Provencal Soup - pg. 268
- Avocado and Roesti Salad - pg. 269

CHAPTER TEN

- Curing Olives - pg. 276
- Popcorn and Mixed Nut Brittle - pg. 277
- Augustina's Jollof Rice - pg. 284
- Basic Cornbread - pg. 286
- Making Jam - pg. 289
- Melon and Orange Jam - pg. 291
- Orange Marmalade - pg. 291
- Fresh Mint Chutney - pg. 297
- Candied Peel - pg. 298

CHAPTER ELEVEN

- Honeycomb - pg. 320
- Nougat - pg. 326
- Hot and Spicy Banana Ketchup - pg. 337
- Mum's Relish - pg. 338
- Shane's Mango Sauce - pg. 339

Dear Gus' <u>Rich Fruit Cake</u>

1 lb Raisins (seeded)
8 ozs (chopped almonds)
8 ozs (glace cherries)
8 ozs (mixed peel)
1½ sultanas
½ currants
⅔ cup brandy or (orange juice)
20 ozs plain flour & 4 ozs S.R. Flour
½ teas salt
1 teas grated nutmeg
1 teas cinnamon
2 teas mixed spice
1 lb butter
1 lb brown sugar
4 tables marmalade (or dark jam)
2 teas vanilla essence.
8 eggs.

Cook 4 hrs (2 hrs for half mixture)

Mix butter & sugar till creamy add eggs one at a time then flour & fruit alternately

Hope this will be the start to your success in life.
Love Nanna.

Printed in Australia
AUHW010812170220
323821AU00008BA/8

9 780648 782100